S0-ADM-779

ULCERS

ULCERS

A GUIDE TO DIAGNOSIS,
TREATMENT AND PREVENTION

Ricki Ostrov

Thorsons
An Imprint of HarperCollins*Publishers*

Thorsons
An Imprint of HarperCollins*Publishers*
77–85 Fulham Palace Road,
Hammersmith, London W6 8JB
1160 Battery Street,
San Francisco, California 94111–1213

Published by Thorsons 1996

1 3 5 7 9 10 8 6 4 2

© Ricki Ostrov 1996

Ricki Ostrov asserts the moral right to
be identified as the author of this work

A catalogue record for this book
is available from the British Library

ISBN 0 7225 3252 0

Printed and bound in Great Britain by
Caledonian International Book Manufacturing Ltd, Glasgow

All rights reserved. No part of this publication may be
reproduced, stored in a retrieval system, or transmitted,
in any form or by any means, electronic, mechanical,
photocopying, recording or otherwise, without the prior
permission of the publishers.

CONTENTS

ACKNOWLEDGEMENTS

The author would like to extend special thanks to Dr Steven Moss.

FOREWORD

Peptic ulcers of the stomach and duodenum continue to be a major medical problem. They cause severe pain and indigestion in perhaps 10 per cent of people at some stage in their life, and even today cause premature death due to complications of haemorrhage or bleeding.

Ricki Ostrov has prepared a detailed and authoritative account of the scientific background to the development of peptic ulceration, and the recent major changes in the way that patients with peptic ulcers can be treated.

Until 1976, the only definitive treatment was for the peptic ulcer patient to undergo some form of surgical procedure to control the stomach's ability to secrete acid. These operations were not always successful, and they often left the patient a gastric cripple, unable to eat normal meals.

Twenty years ago British researchers discovered a new class of drugs (the histamine H_2-receptor antagonists) that transformed the lives of patients with peptic ulceration. The tablets controlled gastric acid secretion, and rapidly relieved all symptoms. However, patients were soon symptomatic again unless they continued taking a low dose of the drug each night.

Ten years ago a new bacterium was discovered – *Helicobacter pylori*. It was found that this bacterium was a vital co-factor in the development of peptic ulcer. Treatment with a suitable combination of antibiotics can sterilize the lining of the stomach and eradicate infection with the bacterium, resulting in a permanent cure of peptic ulceration.

This book provides the opportunity for patients with peptic ulceration to understand their disease. It explains the processes of digestion, mechanisms by which ulcers occur, the symptoms of ulcer disease, and the techniques used to investigate the upper digestive tract. It explains the advantages and disadvantages of different forms of treatment for peptic ulceration using both the drugs of modern medicine and also simple changes to lifestyle that may help. Informed patients can face their peptic ulcer with confidence – now that effective medical treatment is available for everybody.

RE Pounder, MA MD DSc (Med) FRCP
Professor of Medicine
Royal Free Hospital and School of Medicine
Hampstead, London

INTRODUCTION

It is estimated that between 5 and 10 per cent of the population will suffer a peptic ulcer at some time in their lives. It is more likely to occur as you get older, and tends to affect slightly more men than women.

Peptic ulcers are often considered a minor condition by patients. They start to feel that burning sensation and pop a few antacid tablets or drink a glass of milk. What they fail to realize is that peptic ulcers can become a very serious condition.

In Britain, peptic ulcers account for almost 60,000 hospital admissions each year. Over 4,500 people die from complications of ulcers, such as bleeding or perforation. This is more than twice the number of women who die from cervical cancer.

In the past doctors had little to offer sufferers of ulcers except for antacids, and if these failed, surgery. But a revolution occurred in the mid-1970s with the development of a new type of drug called H_2 antagonists. As a result, many fewer patients needed surgery and ulcers could be continuously healed, although not necessarily cured.

An even more recent discovery concerns the importance of a tiny bacterium called *Helicobacter pylori*, which has again dramatically changed the treatment of ulcer disease. As doctors are finding out more about the role of *H. pylori*, it appears that finally many ulcers can be cured once and for all rather than simply being kept under control.

Understanding and knowledge about peptic ulcers are changing rapidly, and it is likely that within the next few years we will see a revolution in the way they are treated.

This book aims to help you understand what an ulcer is, why it develops, and what you can do about it.

Chapter 1 explains how your digestive system works. Without this knowledge it would be difficult to understand why ulcers develop. An understanding of this process also helps you to understand the treatments that have been developed for ulcers, and why and how they are effective.

Chapter 2 tells you all about ulcers – what they are, the two types of peptic ulcers, what causes ulcers, and the symptoms. With this information you will be able to understand what your doctor is telling you about your condition. It also helps to explain the symptoms you may be suffering, and specifically about the type of ulcer you have developed.

Chapter 3 covers *Helicobacter pylori*, the bacterium now thought to be responsible for the majority of ulcers. The story of its discovery, how it affects your stomach and duodenum, and how it causes ulcers to develop are all explained here.

Chapter 4 explains the risk factors for developing a peptic ulcer. Even though you may be infected with *Helicobacter pylori*, so are millions of others who do not go on to develop ulcers. This may help to explain why other factors, for instance cigarette smoking, your sex and age, your diet and even your blood group may have a role to play.

Chapter 5 tells you what to expect when seeing your GP, which will undoubtedly be your first port of call. Although each patient/doctor relationship is different, there are general assumptions on the best way of diagnosing and treating peptic ulcer disease. This helps you understand why your doctor might examine you and ask certain questions about your health and lifestyle, and what to expect from your initial consultations.

Chapter 6 explains how a peptic ulcer is diagnosed. There are two ways of doing this – a barium meal X-ray or endoscopy. Both investigations are clearly explained so you will know why one test is chosen over another, what will happen before, during and after the investigation, and what type of information will be gleaned from the results.

Chapter 7 covers the treatments for peptic ulcers, including antacids, H_2 antagonists and proton pump inhibitors. It details the doses, effectiveness and side-effects of the various medications, and also explains what might occur if the treatment is unsuccessful or if you have a relapse. This chapter also explains eradication therapy (treatment to eliminate *Helicobacter pylori*) and why it has caused so much excitement in the medical world.

Chapter 8 provides information on the dangers of ulcers, including bleeding and perforation. It explains what these conditions are, why they occur, and the treatments used for curing them. You will understand the different types of surgery, which type is currently most popular and most common, and what to expect in terms of relief and recovery.

Chapter 9 will tell you how you can help yourself. It provides information on diet and lifestyle changes you can make to improve your overall health, such as how to reduce stress and use complementary therapies in addition to any medical treatment to improve your health and well-being.

At the end of the book are useful addresses and phone numbers of organizations to contact to find out more about treatment or about peptic ulcer disease in general.

Although the treatment of peptic ulcers is constantly changing, there is little doubt that a revolution has occurred with the discovery of *Helicobacter pylori*. If you are an ulcer sufferer, by understanding as much as you can about your condition you will hopefully be able to make the necessary changes so that you are never troubled by an ulcer again.

1

THE DIGESTIVE PROCESS

There are a number of different mechanisms that take place in the stomach and intestine, and many of these will in turn affect whether or not you develop an ulcer. Learning about these mechanisms will help you to understand the various treatments used for peptic ulcers and how they work.

Although the digestive process may at first sound pretty simple and straightforward, there are lots of different things that can go wrong. When they do, they can lead to a host of digestive troubles such as indigestion (dyspepsia) and, of course, ulcers.

The Digestive Tract

The digestive system, or gastrointestinal tract, begins at your mouth and ends at your anus. It is similar to one long tube which varies in size, structure and function all along the way. Most of this tube has layers of muscles lining its walls which squeeze the food along in a rhythmic process called peristalsis.

In various places along the digestive tract there are rings of muscles called sphincter muscles. The role of the sphincter muscles is to allow only small amounts of food to be sent on at a time. They also help to prevent partially-digested matter to re-enter the previous part of the digestive tract.

For example, there are sphincter muscles at the bottom end of the oesophagus. When food enters the stomach these muscles become tightly closed. This helps keep the contents of the stomach from backing up, a condition called reflux or regurgitation.

The first part of the gastrointestinal tract is the mouth. It is here that the digestive process begins. By chewing food you break it down into more manageable parts. This process is aided by saliva, the secretions from the salivary glands.

Next comes the oesophagus. This is the muscular tube that carries food from the throat to the stomach.

It is in the stomach that the main digestive processes start. The stomach is like a reservoir, designed to hold food for several hours until the small intestine is ready for it. It allows the rest of the gut to cope with a large meal by sending down partially-digested food a little at a time.

The stomach is divided into two sections. The antrum is the lower third of the stomach. This is where most of the hormonal activity necessary for digestion takes place. It is in the antrum that instructions are given to the rest of the stomach to start producing its acid and pepsin to help digest and sterilize the food.

At the lower end of the stomach is a muscular valve called the pylorus. It is through the pylorus that food is moved into the small intestine, a long coiled tube about 6 metres (18 ft) long. It is called the small intestine because of its small diameter, not because of its length — it is actually longer than the large intestine. The small intestine consists of three sections: the duodenum (the uppermost part of the small intestine), the jejunum, and the ileum. The digestive process continues all along the small intestine, and nutrients are absorbed into the cells which line the tract.

The small intestine leads on to the large intestine, or colon. This is wider than the small intestine, but shorter – about 2 m (6 ft) in length. It is here that water and salts from digested material are reabsorbed back into your system.

The last section of the digestive tract is the rectum. It is here that waste matter is stored and eventually expelled as faeces through the anus.

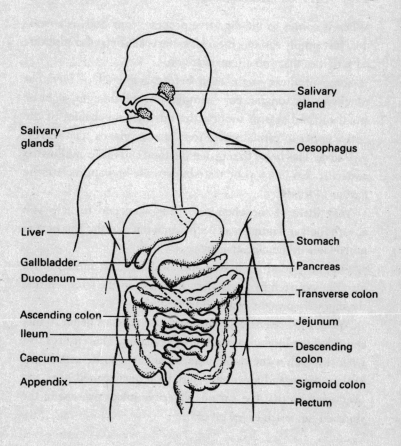

Salivary gland

Salivary glands

Oesophagus

Liver

Stomach

Gallbladder

Pancreas

Duodenum

Transverse colon

Ascending colon

Jejunum

Ileum

Descending colon

Caecum

Appendix

Sigmoid colon

Rectum

The Digestive Tract

Even though a great deal of activity is taking place, you'll feel very little – if any – of this. That is because the digestive process is controlled by the autonomic (involuntary) nervous system. This regulates the peristaltic action of the muscles and the production of the digestive enzymes and hormones.

The Start of the Process

When it comes to the digestive process, your body is a wonder. Just simply eating a meal kick-starts all sorts of complicated activities that you are unaware of.

Some of these begin even before a morsel of food has touched your tongue. For example, just the thought, sight or smell of food sets in motion the intricate mechanics of the entire upper intestinal tract. Your salivary glands start secreting saliva. This helps to moisten the food and make swallowing easier. It also helps your taste buds sense and appreciate the flavour of foods.

Very little of the chemical changes needed to help you absorb food and nutrients take place in the mouth. This occurs much later in the digestive process.

Once the food is chewed and swallowed, it moves down into the stomach by peristalsis. It is here in the stomach that the digestive process well and truly starts.

When food reaches the stomach, the muscles begin to mix and grind the food into much smaller matter. This ensures that when it reaches the duodenum it can start to be more fully broken down and absorbed. The food gets turned over and over again so that the various digestive juices present in the stomach can reach every bit of it.

THREE KEY SUBSTANCES

The walls of the stomach are rich in glands which secrete three substances that play a major role in the digestive process. These substances also have a vital role to play in the development of peptic ulcers.

1 **Hydrochloric acid** is secreted by parietal cells. These are special cells located in the lining of the stomach, or the mucosa. Men have about one thousand million parietal cells; women have about 800 million. The parietal cells are located in the top two-thirds of the stomach – there are no parietal cells in the antrum. The presence of hydrochloric acid helps to create the environment essential if the digestive enzymes are to work effectively. At the same time hydrochloric acid disinfects food, destroying most harmful bacteria that might be present.

2 A group of digestive enzymes called **pepsins** are also secreted by the stomach mucosa. It is the pepsin cells, called the chief cells, which are responsible for the secretion of pepsin. Pepsin can only be secreted when hydrochloric acid is also present. The process is a little complicated. When acid is present in the stomach, a chemical called pepsinogen is secreted. And when pepsinogen, called a pre-cursor to pepsin, comes into contact with acid, the pepsinogen turns into pepsin. The job of the pepsin enzymes is to break down proteins in the food into small chains of amino acids so they can be absorbed further down in the small intestine.

3 When a meal arrives from the mouth to the stomach, powerful hormones called **gastrins** start to be secreted directly into the bloodstream. A type of cell, the G cell, is responsible for this. And G cells are only located in the antrum, the bottom third of the stomach.

The job of gastrins is to keep the flow of gastric juice high and also to start off the secretion of pepsin and acid. They keep the gastric juice at a very high level until the entire meal is digested.

This process works like a feedback loop. Other cells near the G cells produce a hormone called somatostatin. Somatostatin can only send its messages a very short distance — about a few millimetres. It does not act through the bloodstream. It works to alert other cells to trigger or stop production of their hormones and secretions. And so it is somatostatin that tells the G cells what to do. If somatostatin is present, the production of gastrin is decreased. If somatostatin is inhibited, the production of gastrin is increased.

When gastrin is secreted, it enters the bloodstream and eventually flows back to the stomach. It is only when it reaches the stomach via the bloodstream that it stimulates the outpouring of gastric juice and acids.

The stomach mucosa is lined with a single layer of cells that produce and secrete a jelly-like mucus. This helps protect the stomach from the harsh effects of hydrochloric acid and pepsin. If there was not some sort of defensive layer in the stomach, it would end up digesting itself. This inner surface of the stomach wall, the gastric mucosa, contains millions of cells that, as with other cells, are continuously being sloughed off and replaced. The stomach mucosa replaces itself about once every three days.

The Role of the Vagus Nerve

Your stomach works 24 hours a day. Even at night, while you are sleeping, your body's secretory mechanisms continue to work, although at very low levels. This means that your stomach is always ready to digest a meal, should one appear.

This is why even the sight or smell of food can get your digestive juices flowing. The brain switches on the vagus nerve, which runs from the brain through the neck, alongside your oesophagus, to the stomach. The vagus nerve is responsible for the secretion of digestive acid. It carries the command from the brain to the stomach, and directly to the pepsin and parietal cells, to start pouring out their products. It also helps control stomach movements, or motility.

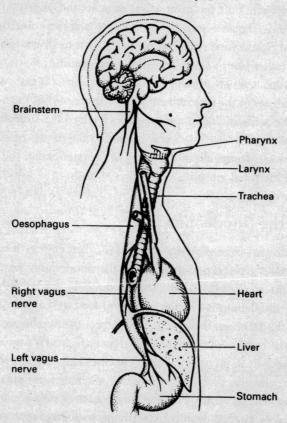

The Route of the Vagus Nerve

There are a number of different safety features in the digestive process. If these did not work, your stomach would be in a constant state of producing and secreting acids, even though they were not needed.

As your appetite begins to be satisfied, the vagus nerve stops sending instructions from the brain to the stomach. And as the stomach starts emptying itself of both the solid and liquid parts of the meal, the pressure on the stomach wall decreases. This means that your stomach will begin to feel less full, and will stop triggering off the production of acids and juices. At the same time, the acid secreted by the stomach runs over the G cell and turns off its chemical message. This feedback process works rather like an automatic pilot or thermostat.

Another safety feature in the digestive process is that, when the contents of the stomach enters the upper part of the intestine, the acids and fats send messages back to the stomach to slow down. This signal is accomplished by the release of several hormones from cells in the lining of the duodenum, the first part of the small intestine.

Into the Duodenum

Food that has been partially digested is called chyme. It is this that passes from the stomach into the duodenum, which is about 30 cm (12 in) long and shaped similarly to a horseshoe.

The duodenum is the meeting point for three organs – the stomach, the common bile duct (which contributes bile secreted by the liver), and the pancreatic duct (which adds pancreatic enzymes to the mixture). These enzymes help digest protein and fat, and also provide an alkaline-containing bicarbonate in fluid form. This bicarb, just like bicarbonate of soda you might use in your kitchen or in cooking, helps to neutralize the acids that have passed from the stomach. Bile and the pancreatic enzymes are also strongly alkaline. This further helps to neutralize the strongly acidic chyme, and by so doing helps to protect the duodenum from ulceration and inflammation.

This neutralizing of the stomach contents is a complicated process. It is made possible by the working of certain hormones, also known as the body's chemical messengers.

When the duodenum detects the presence of acid and some amino acids, it releases two hormones into your bloodstream. The first, secretin, sends a message to the pancreas to pour out water and bicarbonate of soda. It also tells the stomach to stop making and secreting acid.

The second hormone, cholecystokinin, signals the pancreas to pour out and send along the three major groups of digestive enzymes. At the same time, cholecystokinin stimulates the gallbladder to contract and pass its bile down the common bile duct into the duodenum. Bile acts like a detergent, breaking up fat into droplets.

So the duodenum releases chemical messengers which, via the bloodstream, return to the stomach. These tell the stomach to slow down the secretion of acids, and signal the gallbladder and pancreas to add their digestive enzymes to the meal, which is still being moved along the small intestine by waves of peristalsis (muscular contractions).

The Role of the Small Intestine

In the small intestine, almost all of the contents of our food and drink are absorbed after being broken down into their constituent parts. It is also here that the fluids poured into the intestine by its own secretions are absorbed back into the body.

It is a big job for the small intestine. If you add up all the saliva, gastric acid secretions, bile and pancreatic juice, plus fluid secreted by the intestinal cells, the result is 9 or 10 litres

(8 or 9 quarts) of water and salts moved down the intestine each day. And about nine-tenths of this is reabsorbed lower down in the intestine.

This process, which may sound time-consuming, actually happens very quickly. The partially-digested stomach contents begin to leave the stomach promptly – almost half of a meal has left about and hour and half after you've eaten it, and almost all of it is gone from the stomach three hours after eating, depending in part on its fat content.

The major portion of the meal moves from the duodenum into the first portion of the large intestine at different speeds in different individuals. In some it can get there in 90 minutes; in others the meal moves much more slowly and may take three or four hours. This has little to do with the health of your digestive tract, and more to do with what you've eaten. Carbohydrates and protein are quickly absorbed from the jejunum, while fats take a little bit longer.

The stomach and the duodenum are concerned with the digestion, or breaking down of food. Absorption of waters and nutrients into the bloodstream takes place primarily in the jejunum and the ileum. It is here that the tiny molecules that arise from the breakdown of proteins, carbohydrates and fats, including vitamins and water, enter the cells lining the small intestine. From the small intestine they are sent around the body via the bloodstream and the lymph vessels.

After all of this has taken place the leftover residue is squeezed into the large intestine, where 90 per cent of the water is reabsorbed. The remainder is stored in the rectum and eventually expelled through the anus. The entire process, from the first morsel to the final bowel movement, can take around two to three days.

2

ALL ABOUT ULCERS

Although the stomach normally has efficient mechanisms for neutralizing and diluting harsh stomach chemicals and acid, a number of things can go wrong with this process. And when something does go wrong, the result can be a peptic ulcer.

An ulcer is a crater in the tissue covering one of the surfaces of the body, or one of the protective mucous membranes that line many parts of the body, including the digestive tract. You can get an ulcer almost anywhere, for example in the skin, the cornea of the eye, the lining of the mouth or the lining of various parts of the digestive tract.

What Are Peptic Ulcers?

The term 'peptic ulcer' refers to ulcers that occur as a result of the action of pepsin and acid on the mucous lining. There are two types of peptic ulcers: stomach ulcers, which are often referred to as gastric ulcers, and duodenal ulcers, which occur in the duodenum (the uppermost part of the small intestine near the stomach).

Peptic ulcers develop when pepsin and acids break through the protective lining of the stomach or duodenum and eat into the underlying tissues. Normally the stomach lining (the mucosa) provides protection against the harsh actions of pepsin and hydrochloric acid. But if the lining becomes weakened for some reason, it actually digests a part of itself, causing a crater or hole. The result is a peptic ulcer. True peptic ulcers extend deeply, through the entire thickness of the mucosal lining. Shallow defects that do not do this are called erosions.

Peptic ulcers tend to be round or oval, but occasionally they have an irregular or linear shape. They can vary widely in size, from a few millimetres to a few centimetres. However, most are smaller than 2 cm (1 inch) in diameter. In most cases ulcers occur singly. However, in a few cases a person may have two or three at the same time.

What Goes Wrong with Ulcers?

The two harsh ingredients, hydrochloric acid and pepsin, must be present together to cause an ulcer. Pepsin, without acid, will not do any damage.

But how does this mechanism work? It would seem likely that a person who produces too much acid will develop an ulcer. But this is not always the case. Gastric ulcer sufferers do not always make more acid than non-sufferers. And though the majority of patients with duodenal ulcers do produce more acid than is normal, this again is not true in every case. So too much acid cannot be the whole story.

Instead of simply being the result of too much acid, ulcers develop when there is a breakdown in the balance between the acid/pepsin levels and the normal protective mechanisms in the stomach wall.

How the Stomach Protects Itself

Normally the stomach and duodenum are well protected from the harsh effects of pepsin and acids. There are a number of ways this is accomplished.

- The surface lining cells produce a thick layer of mucus that coats the stomach wall. This keeps the acids and pepsin at bay.
- The cells in the stomach lining also pour forth their own natural antacid, bicarbonate of soda, which helps to neutralize stomach acid.
- If the pepsin and acid break through and an injury does take place, the neighbouring surface cells go to work to fill the gap and replace damaged cells.
- Prostaglandins (chemical substances in the stomach lining) help to provide protection by increasing the blood flow to the troubled areas. They also help to increase the amounts of bicarbonate and mucus produced.

The Two Types of Ulcers

As mentioned earlier, there are two types of peptic ulcers: stomach (gastric) ulcers, and duodenal ulcers.

WHO GETS DUODENAL ULCERS?

Duodenal ulcers are by far the most common type of peptic ulcer. They are about twice as common in men as in women, although in many parts of the Western world duodenal ulcers are becoming less common in men but more so among women.

In men, duodenal ulcers occur much earlier in life than gastric ulcers, usually from around the age of 25 onwards, with the peak age being 45 years. Women, however, develop duodenal ulcers later, usually beginning around the age of 45. Unlike gastric ulcers, duodenal ulcers are almost never malignant (cancerous).

In the 19th century, gastric ulcers were much more common than duodenal ulcers. But in the 20th century a change has taken place, and duodenal ulcers have overtaken gastric ulcers. Overall, however, since the 1950s there seems to have been a decline in the rate of duodenal ulcers in Western countries such as Great Britain and the United States.

There are also regional differences. In the UK, for instance, duodenal ulcers become more common the further north you travel. There is a higher rate in Scotland than there is in the southeast of England.

Another interesting fact is that people with blood group O are slightly more likely to develop a duodenal ulcer. It is thought that people in this blood group produce more parietal cells than people in other blood groups. You are also more at risk of duodenal ulcer if a first-degree relative (mother, father or siblings) also has (or has had) one.

WHO GETS STOMACH ULCERS?

Stomach ulcers are about four times less common than duodenal ulcers. They often occur later in life and, unlike duodenal ulcers, can occasionally be malignant (cancerous). Males are slightly more affected than females, and the peak incidence occurs between the ages of around 55 and 65 years of age.

Interestingly, there is a slightly greater increase in incidence in people who are of the blood group A. As with duodenal ulcers, there is also an increased incidence if a first-degree relative suffers with a stomach ulcer. And stomach ulcers are more common in certain countries, for instance Japan and Peru, than in others.

It used to be thought that stomach ulcers were more likely to affect people in semi-skilled and unskilled professions, while duodenal ulcers affected the more professional classes. There seems to be little truth to this theory. In recent data from both Britain and the US, it appears that both types of ulcers are more common among people lower down the socio-economic scale.

How Do You Know It's an Ulcer?

In most cases ulcers cause very clear symptoms, though a small percentage of people suffer from 'silent ulcers' (*see page 20*) which cause no obvious symptoms such as pain or indigestion, but can result in serious complications if left untreated.

The classic symptom and most common complaint is pain centred in the epigastric area. This is pain in the central upper abdomen, just under the rib cage. Some studies have shown that pain affects almost all patients. Others put the figure at 70 per cent of patients with duodenal ulcers, and about 50 per cent of those with stomach ulcers.

Many doctors hear patients describe the terrible pain of ulcers as a burning sensation, or a feeling of constant hunger. They may also say they have a sensation of pressure in the area.

An acute attack of ulcer pain can last from around 30 minutes to a couple of hours. It is hard to be specific, as so many sufferers will eat something or take antacids to relieve the pain quickly. This makes it difficult for doctors to be precise about the length of a 'normal' attack of ulcer pain.

The pain may be felt over a wide area. In about 60 per cent of people it radiates and spreads to other areas, most commonly the back and other parts of the abdomen. However, when patients see their doctors they are often able to pinpoint the area where they experience most pain.

It's also common for the pain, or attacks, to come and go over a period of time. You may find you go through a few days or a week experiencing episodes of terrific pain and discomfort, then these go away for quite a while, somewhere between a month and six months.

During an attack the pain is rarely constant. You may find that it fluctuates in intensity, and you'll also have pain-free intervals. In some cases food may relieve the pain, or make it worse, or even have no effect at all. The pain will also have some distinguishing features, depending on the type of ulcer you have.

Case Study – Pain

The pain I get with my ulcer is different than any other pain I've ever had. It's similar to a burning ache, right in the centre of my abdomen below the breast area. It's just so much worse than anything I've ever experienced. It's terrible.

I have to admit I drink a lot of coffee, at least five or six cups in the morning and then continue all through the day. I've noticed that when my ulcer is acting up, if I cut back it really makes a difference. And though I like to have a few drinks on the weekend, this really kills my ulcer. It's just not worth it, and even taking an extra dose of medication won't help with this.

I usually get some warning signs even before my ulcer comes back. For about two weeks beforehand I seem to feel constantly nauseous, and have a gnawing sensation in the pit of my stomach. It doesn't seem to make a difference if I've eaten something or not, the feeling just seems to sit there.

Then the pain starts up. And when it hurts, it's terrible. Sometimes it's so bad it wakes me up in the middle of the night. I usually try to catch it before it gets this far and I start taking my Zantac again. But even if I get woken up, I find drinking a glass of milk seems to help a lot and calm it down.

I've started to watch what I eat and drink, to see if changing my diet will help at all. And I find that if I avoid eating large meals this seems to reduce the amount of pain. I don't know if there's any scientific evidence for this. But it makes a real difference to how I feel.

CARL, 38

DUODENAL ULCERS

If you have a duodenal ulcer, it's more likely you will experience pain than if you had a stomach ulcer. It usually begins to occur around one to three hours after you've eaten a meal. And you may find that the pain comes back again in the middle of the night, often between 1 and 3 a.m., and wakes you up. This is probably because the stomach is empty of food, so there is nothing in the stomach to buffer the effects of the acid that is constantly being produced in readiness for a meal.

Ironically, when your stomach is empty there is less acid present, but the acidity, or pH balance, is highest. When you have food in your stomach you are producing much more acid – about four times more acid per minute than when the stomach is empty – but this acid is 'watered down' by the presence of food and drink.

Compared with a stomach ulcer, it's more common that the pain of a duodenal ulcer can be relieved by eating something, drinking milk or taking antacids. It's also often easier to pinpoint the exact site of the pain. And patients with duodenal ulcers have usually suffered pain for a long period of time, on and off for many years.

There are other symptoms that may accompany a duodenal ulcer. These most commonly include nausea, vomiting, weight loss or some bleeding in the stools.

STOMACH ULCERS

There are several contrasts between stomach and duodenal ulcers. Pain is a symptom in only about half of all people with stomach ulcers, although it is usually located in the same area as in the case of a duodenal ulcer. Less frequently the pain can be relieved by eating something, drinking milk or taking some over-the-counter antacids. But the relief they provide is often short lived. The pain usually returns with a vengeance about 30 minutes after a meal, though in some cases you'll be pain-free for a couple of hours after eating. Some patients with gastric ulcers may find, however, that eating makes their pain worse.

Gastric ulcers are less often accompanied by other symptoms such as nausea and vomiting. However, loss of appetite is twice as common in gastric ulcer patients as in those with a duodenal ulcer. It occurs in approximately two thirds of those with gastric ulcers. If, therefore, you suffer daily pain brought on by eating and accompanied by loss of appetite, you probably have a stomach ulcer rather than a duodenal ulcer.

People suffering from gastric ulcers often go to the doctor sooner than patients with duodenal ulcers, after having suffered for a shorter period of time – less than a year.

Why Does It Hurt?

Not much is known about why ulcers are painful. It is thought the pain comes from the ulcer itself, and that acid irritates the open sore, especially in duodenal ulcer pain.

It is generally accepted that stomach acid is the key factor in causing the pain. This is why, when you eat something, especially protein foods, the food helps to provide a buffer against the effects of acid, neutralizing them.

The pain usually returns a few hours after eating, because the buffering effect of the food is gone but acid production continues, providing the trigger for pain.

Because the stomach secretes acid 24 hours a day, this could be why nighttime pain is so common with duodenal ulcers. Although there is no food in the stomach, the acid is still present, aggravating the ulcer.

Ulcer Symptoms

- Pain felt high in the centre of the abdomen. It can range from a mild ache to severe discomfort.
- The pain may come on soon after a meal – anywhere from 30 minutes to a couple of hours afterwards.
- Eating something, taking antacids or drinking milk seems to help, though the pain usually returns fairly quickly.
- With duodenal ulcers, the pain may come on at night, waking you up.
- Nausea and vomiting may be present, though more commonly in duodenal ulcers than stomach ulcers. Vomiting may relieve some of the pain.
- You may lose weight for no apparent reason.
- The attacks may last for some days, then fade for weeks or months before recurring.
- Silent, or symptomless ulcers, may lead to bleeding. This is characterized by vomiting blood or passing black, tarry stools.

Silent Ulcers

Sometimes peptic ulcers do not cause any pain. They are then referred to as 'silent ulcers', and most commonly occur in people who have been taking drugs such as NSAIDs (non-steroidal anti-inflammatory drugs) for chronic conditions such as arthritis or rheumatism. These pain-killers can mask the pain of an ulcer.

Silent ulcers can persist for some time without causing any problems. However, one of the big dangers with silent ulcers is that, without treatment, they cause serious complications such as bleeding and perforation. Many people first go to their doctor because they have noticed signs of this kind of complication rather than because they have noticed the more classic symptoms of an ulcer.

Bleeding from an ulcer occurs when the ulcer has broken through a blood vessel in the stomach or duodenum. It usually causes vomiting of blood or the passage of black, tar-like stools. Sometimes the bleeding is slow and hidden ('occult'), causing iron-deficiency anaemia.

Perforation, which is more common with duodenal than gastric ulcers, occurs when the ulcer has gone so deep it eats through the entire thickness of the wall of the duodenum or stomach. This can allow the contents of these organs to leak into the abdomen, causing infection and inflammation – a condition known as peritonitis.

Both bleeding and perforation are considered to be medical emergencies. These are serious complications, and if not treated immediately can be fatal.

Another danger of silent ulcers is a much rarer condition called pyloric stenosis. This can occur due to a thickening and scarring of the pylorus, the muscular valve linking the stomach to the duodenum. If stenosis occurs, it can prevent food from moving from the stomach into the small intestine, leading to constipation, vomiting and abdominal discomfort. *(For more information see Chapter 8.)*

3

THE ULCER BUG

In the past 15 years there has been a revolution in the thinking about peptic ulcers. There have been so many unanswered questions about the disease, for instance why it has such a high recurrence rate, why some people are so much more susceptible than others, and why ulcers seem to run in families.

The discovery of the role of a bacterium called *Helicobacter pylori* may be the key to finding the answers to these questions and many others. And this new information about *H. pylori* has radically altered the treatment of the disease.

What Is *Helicobacter Pylori*?

Helicobacter pylori was probably first observed as early as 1906. Because its significance was not understood, the bacterium now called *H. pylori* was essentially forgotten until the early 1980s, when its importance was discovered by Australian doctors.

H. pylori is a spiral-shaped bacterium found in the stomach. Initially it was thought to be similar to the Campylobacter group of bacteria. As a result it was first called *Campylobacter pylori*. Then by 1989 it was determined that it was not a true campylobacter, and was reclassified and renamed *Helicobacter pylori* because it has a helical, or spiral, shape.

H. pylori is found in the mucous layer of the stomach and the duodenum, though it definitely seems to prefer the stomach lining, finding the environment there extremely favourable. It seems to stick only to gastric cells in the stomach lining, and in fact usually only affects the duodenum when there is a change in the cells, called metaplasia, in which they begin to resemble stomach cells.

HOW IT WAS FOUND

When reading about the 'rediscovery' of *Helicobacter pylori*, it sounds like a medical mystery story.

The heroes of this story are Drs Barry Marshall and Robin Warren from Australia. In 1982 they discovered the spiral-shaped bacteria in the stomach of almost all of their patients brought in for endoscopy (an examination of the stomach and duodenum using the fibre-optic endoscope, a telescope-like instrument). When examining the biopsy specimens from about 100 consecutive patients with chronic gastritis, or inflammation of the stomach lining, they kept finding evidence of the presence of the bacterium. Although initially this seemed unlikely, as it was at that time assumed nothing could survive in the harsh, acidic conditions of the stomach. But the doctors persisted in investigating their finding.

First they cultured the organism in the laboratory. This was the first known culture of *Helicobacter pylori* and the first time that the bacterium's association with chronic gastritis was described. After closely studying *H. pylori*'s effect on the stomach, they then proposed that this bacterium was the underlying cause of both gastritis and peptic ulcers. They came to this conclusion because all of their patients with duodenal ulcers, and 80 per cent of the patients with stomach ulcers, were infected with the bacteria. The remaining 20 per cent had been taking NSAIDs (non-steroidal anti-inflammatory drugs) such as aspirin or ibuprofen, a common and known cause of stomach ulcers.

Drs Marshall and Warren wrote up their findings, and the landmark study was published in *The Lancet* in 1984.[1] Their conclusion caused an absolute uproar within the medical profession, and was hotly debated and disputed around the globe.

To prove they were right, Dr Barry Marshall decided to perform an experiment. He actually infected himself with *H. pylori*, and a few days later developed symptoms of gastritis, such as nausea, bad breath and indigestion – symptoms he had never experienced before.

In spite of the initial scepticism and reluctance to accept *H. pylori*'s role in ulcers, studies and evidence linking the two have mounted. Hundreds of studies from around the world have confirmed its presence in most people with ulcers. Many medical experts have done studies and come to the same conclusion about the connection between *H. pylori* and peptic ulcers.

A number of other studies, again many by Dr Marshall, proved that when you eradicate *H. pylori*, the ulcer goes away and doesn't come back. This evidence is what convinced a lot of doctors of the importance of *H. pylori* in peptic ulcer disease.

ITS ROLE IN ULCER DISEASE

Although doctors were finally beginning to accept *H. pylori*'s role in ulcer disease, what the studies did not explain was the link between the two, and exactly how *H. pylori* could cause ulcers. So the next step was to try to find out the exact mechanism that comes into play. There are a number of theories about this, and still much disagreement in the medical world.

Initially it was suspected that *H. pylori* increased the output of acid in the stomach. However, studies have not been able to prove this conclusively. In fact, many studies have shown that patients with *H. pylori* infection and ulcers have normal or even below-normal levels of acid production. Alternative explanations were needed.

A great deal of research is taking place to determine the effects of *Helicobacter pylori*. Scientists believe that, because of the special shape of the bacterium and its specific characteristics, it works to damage the stomach and duodenal tissue in a number of ways, leading to the development of ulcers.

Altering the Acid/Alkaline Balance

The amazing thing about *H. pylori*, and the reason some doctors were so reluctant to accept its role, is that it was previously thought that no bacterium (nor anything else) could survive in the harsh, hostile, acidic environment of the stomach.

Studies have found that *H. pylori* can and does survive because it produces large quantities of the enzyme urease. Urease, in turn, converts the urea present in stomach juices into bicarbonate and ammonia. These substances work together to neutralize stomach acids, and cause the stomach to become an alkaline environment, extremely suitable for the survival of the bacteria.

Another effect of making the stomach environment more alkaline is that *H. pylori* destroys the structure of the protective mucous layer. This allows the bacteria to migrate into the less acidic mucus of the stomach lining, or even beneath the mucous lining. It finds itself a handy little niche that is safe from the stomach acids. And once *H. pylori* has taken up residence in the mucous lining, it can easily produce more urease.

Damaging the Stomach Lining

Because of their spiral shape and the way they move, the *H. pylori* bacteria have been shown actually to penetrate the stomach's protective mucous lining. Here they can safely produce substances that weaken the stomach's protective mucus and make the stomach cells more susceptible to the damaging effects of acid and pepsin.

The bacteria can also easily attach themselves to stomach cells. This further weakens the stomach's defence mechanism and produces sites of local inflammation.

Sticking to Stomach Cells

Excess stomach acid and other irritating factors cause inflammation of the upper end of the duodenum (the duodenal bulb). In some people, over long periods of time, this inflammation results in the production of stomach-like cells called duodenal gastric metaplasia. Because *H. pylori* is very attracted to stomach cells, it attacks these areas of gastric metaplasia, causing further tissue damage and inflammation, which may result in an ulcer. It's thought that if a person does not have gastric metaplasia, then he or she will not develop a duodenal ulcer.

Causing Inflammation

In areas where there are pockets of *H. pylori* on the lining of the stomach, there is an inflammatory reaction in the cells. These cells become damaged and atrophy, shrinking and dying off. This leads to a thinning of the stomach mucosa. It also diminishes the amount of protective mucus produced, and the amount of bicarbonate of soda secreted from the stomach. When the lining is thinned and less resistant, *H. pylori* somehow digs in and affects the areas of damaged cells. And it seems that it is in these areas that ulcers will develop.

Stimulating Acid Flow

Studies now suggest that *Helicobacter pylori* also stimulates the stomach to produce more acid. It's thought to do this by increasing the circulation and release of gastrin, the hormone released into the blood by cells in the lower end of the stomach. This extra gastrin stimulates the flow of acid from the upper part of the stomach.

H. pylori does this by decreasing the amount of somatostatin that is released onto the neighbouring G cells. And this triggers the G cells to secrete more gastrin and acid.

Releasing Toxins

It's thought that another possible reason *H. pylori* leads to peptic ulcers is that it releases a cytotoxin (poison) which again damages the mucosal lining of the stomach. This may also help produce a better environment for *H. pylori* itself.

However, there are thousands of strains of *H. pylori*, and not all of the strains have toxins. Those that are toxin-free tend not to cause disease. This could be one reason why large numbers of people who are infected with *H. pylori* do not go on to develop ulcers.

TAKEN ALL TOGETHER

Many of the effects of *H. pylori* are closely intertwined. The excess acid may cause inflammation, and this chronic inflammation may damage the lining of the stomach, weakening its protective defence mechanisms. This allows *H. pylori* to set up camp and continue its assault on the stomach lining.

It appears that it is in these weakened areas of tissue that ulcers are more likely to occur. However, this doesn't fully explain why some people with *H. pylori* infection do not go on to develop an ulcer.

It could be that certain strains of *H. pylori* have stronger effects than others, for instance some strains produce toxins and others do not. And scientists do not yet know what is different in those people who develop *H. pylori*-related symptoms or ulcers. Perhaps genetic or environmental factors not yet known make it more likely that some individuals will go on to develop ulcers. All these unanswered questions are the subject of much scientific investigation.

Who Is Affected?

H. pylori infects at least half of the world's population. Until recently it was thought that the infection rates were about the same in men and in women. However, the findings from the largest *H. pylori* prevalence study to date, conducted in Northern Ireland and reported in 1995 at a meeting of the European Helicobacter Pylori Study Group, determined that in Northern Ireland slightly more men than women were infected – just over 52 per cent of men versus 48 per cent of women.

It's thought that infection is transmitted through the faecal-oral route, as is the case with many bacteria. It may also be transmitted from mouth to mouth, as the bacterium has been found in saliva and dental plaque. However, this is not yet proven and is controversial.

The infection rates with *H. pylori* are particularly high in underdeveloped countries. It's suspected that this is due to the lack of public hygiene and sanitation facilities, which makes it easier for cross-infection to occur. And in developing countries the infection seems to be acquired early in life. About 75 per cent of children are infected, and this infection probably remains active for life, as the figures are about the same for adults in the same countries.

In developed countries, however, the picture is somewhat different. Here the infection rates increase with age. For instance, it was assumed that few 10-year-olds are infected — under 5 per cent. However, the Northern Ireland study again found discrepancies. They reported that more than 20 per cent of 12- to 14-year-olds were infected. The rate of infection continues to rise with age. It's estimated that in Britain at least half of all 50-year-olds are infected.

This suggests that each subsequent generation is less likely to become infected, especially during childhood. It may be that improvements in public health, such as cleaner water and better living conditions, are slowly reducing the rate of infection.

There are also differences among ethnic groups and races within the same country. In the US, blacks and Hispanics have higher rates of infection than Caucasians or people of European descent. In Sydney, Australia, there is a higher infection rate among people with Southern European roots than among those who come from an Anglo-Celtic background.

In the UK, studies have shown that infection rates are higher in the lowest social class, and that higher social class groups are less susceptible to infection with *H. pylori* at a young age. This finding was borne out by the Northern Ireland study. Why this occurs isn't known. It's suspected that, again, this may be related to levels of public hygiene.

Another unusual finding from the Northern Ireland study was that infected women were, on average, 1 cm (half an inch) shorter than uninfected women!

H. pylori and Other Conditions

It's now widely accepted that up to 95 per cent of people with duodenal ulcers are infected with *H. pylori*. Of those with stomach ulcers, studies have indicated that somewhere between 70 and 80 per cent have *H. pylori*.

Along with its role in chronic gastritis and peptic ulcers, *Helicobacter pylori* is suspected of playing a part in the development of stomach cancer, and possibly even heart disease.

Stomach cancer is one of the most common malignancies in the world. Studies have shown that *H. pylori* infection is associated with some forms of stomach cancer. And some epidemiological (population) studies have found that gastric cancer occurs more commonly in populations with a higher frequency of *H. pylori* infection. However, gastric cancer does occur in people without infection with *H. pylori*.

As yet, there are no studies that show exactly how *H. pylori* leads to the development of stomach cancer. It's suspected that, because the bacteria causes chronic, almost lifelong gastritis (inflammation of the stomach lining), over the years this leads to damage and changes to the cells lining the stomach. The cells of the stomach proliferate and renew themselves very quickly, unlike some other cells such as brain cells. So these harmful cell changes, called mutations, are reproduced over and over again, eventually creating a tumour. This does not happen overnight. It is more often many years after the initial infection with *H. pylori*.

H. pylori has also been clearly linked with gastric lymphoma, a rare type of stomach cancer. Studies have shown that in some people with the early form of the disease, if you give them radiotherapy and eradication therapy to eliminate the bacteria, the tumour actually goes away.

There's also an interesting theory about a link between *Helicobacter pylori* and heart disease. One study, reported to the British Society of Gastroenterology, found that patients infected with *H. pylori* are almost four times as likely to suffer from heart disease. It's thought that *H. pylori* infection amounts to the same level of risk as smoking 12 to 15 cigarettes a day.

The scientists who reported this link do not know precisely why *H. pylori* could lead to heart disease. Their theory is that the inflammation caused by *H. pylori* raises the level of fibrinogen (a protein found in the blood) and the number of white cells in the blood. These represent major risk factors for heart disease. Many studies are currently underway to try to prove — or disprove – this theory.

Another concern among experts was that *H. pylori* may have a role to play in colon cancer, which is one of the most common cancers in the UK. However, a study published in 1995 found no association between the two whatsoever.[2]

4

THE RISK FACTORS

The discovery of the role of *Helicobacter pylori* has radically altered thinking about the causes of ulcers. In the past there were many misconceptions about the causes of ulcers – many of these perpetuated by the medical profession because so little was known about the disease. Even today, many people still believe that spicy foods or too much stress can cause an ulcer. Studies have consistently shown this to be untrue.

It is now thought that *H. pylori* is the main cause of about 95 per cent of duodenal ulcers, and the culprit in about 75 per cent of gastric ulcers. And yet, although *H. pylori* plays a vital role, it is not the only factor involved in the development of ulcers. Millions of people in the UK are undoubtedly infected with *H. pylori*, but do not go on to develop ulcers. And a number of people without infection do develop ulcers (more often gastric than duodenal ones).

This indicates that other factors play a part in undermining the defence system of the stomach and increasing your risk of an ulcer.

It is now thought that many 'accepted' trigger factors for peptic ulcers may in fact prove to be harmless. Many of the studies were performed before the *H. pylori* connection was discovered, and their findings may eventually prove to be irrelevant. A number of experts and scientists are going back and repeating some of these studies to try once and for all to prove or disprove the link between certain lifestyle factors and peptic ulcer disease.

When you are considering these various trigger factors, you have to separate duodenal from gastric ulcers. Certain factors which may trigger the development of a stomach ulcer have no effect on a duodenal ulcer.

So what does increase your risk? This is where your lifestyle comes into play.

Cigarette Smoking

Although there may not be clear-cut evidence to indicate that certain other factors affect peptic ulcer development, the evidence is fairly concrete when it comes to cigarette smoking. Study after study has repeatedly shown that smoking affects ulcer disease in three ways.

First, it actually increases the incidence of peptic ulcer disease. It's estimated that smokers are twice as likely to develop an ulcer in the first place. And this doesn't just apply to current smokers. Studies have found that people who smoked earlier in life and then gave up are still more likely to develop an ulcer later in life.[1,2]

Second, it slows down the rate of healing. Smokers who have developed an ulcer take longer to heal, even when they are taking strong anti-ulcer medicines and treatment.

Third, cigarette smoking increases your risk of an ulcer recurring after it has been successfully treated. And on a more sombre note, smokers are more likely to die from complications of an ulcer.

These facts are well proven. Furthermore, the frequency

of ulcers increases with the number of cigarettes you smoke. This association with smoking is stronger for men than in women.

WHY DOES THIS OCCUR?

Although the experts know that cigarette smoking affects the progress of ulcer disease, the exact mechanism is still unclear. There are a number of theories as to why this should occur.

An interesting finding to come from the Northern Ireland study discussed earlier is that more smokers than non-smokers were infected with *Helicobacter pylori*. This may provide a clue as to why smokers are more affected than non-smokers by peptic ulcer disease.

It could be that smoking somehow stimulates and increases the acid output in the stomach, but as yet this has not been proven conclusively. It could also be that smoking decreases blood flow to the area. This would impair healing, as it's known that smoking does inhibit wound-healing, for instance after surgery.

Or it could be that smoking reduces the level of protective prostaglandins in the area. It's now thought that smoking interferes with the output of prostaglandins, chemicals which are considered to be important in protecting the upper digestive tract.

All these theories apply to duodenal ulcers. But a little bit more is known about the effect of cigarette smoking on gastric ulcers. It's thought that the nicotine in cigarettes somehow affects the strength of the pyloric sphincter muscle. This is the ring of muscles that surrounds the outlet from the stomach leading to the duodenum. When nicotine causes the pyloric sphincter muscle to weaken, this in turn increases gastroduodenal reflux, allowing harsh bile to flow back into the stomach from the duodenum.

In addition, nicotine reduces bicarbonate secretion from the pancreas. And bicarb is needed to help neutralize the effects of the harsh gastric acid in the duodenum.

Most of the evidence has been gathered on cigarette smokers. As yet there is no evidence either way on whether pipe or cigar smoking is associated with the occurrence of ulcers.

Diet

Contrary to what many people think, your diet seems to have little or no effect on the development of ulcers. What you eat does not seem to cause ulcers and, in spite of anecdotal evidence, even spicy foods do not lead to an ulcer. So far, no studies have proven conclusively that any particular food leads to the development of an ulcer.

One study, in particular, has given spicy foods the all clear.[3] The scientists found that in many areas of India, Malaysia and Africa, where the indigenous populations eat lot of peppers and spicy foods, there is a low incidence of both duodenal and gastric ulcers. So, in theory, spicy foods cannot have any noticeable effect on the development of ulcers. The authors of the study also found conflicting evidence about the effects of peppers on gastric mucosa in both duodenal ulcer patients and healthy volunteers.

Some other studies reported that eating peppers increased acid output, while others reported only a slight increase or none at all. Studies have also shown that red pepper and spices do not damage the gastric mucosa in humans or delay the healing of duodenal ulcers. However, tests on animals did show that whole red peppers damaged the gastric mucosa.

Fibre is another story altogether. There is some evidence that a high-fibre intake seems to be protective against the risk of developing duodenal ulcers. It is thought this could be due to the high levels of carbohydrates in fibre-rich foods, which seem to have a protective effect. Eating a high-fibre diet also seems to reduce the rate of duodenal ulcer recurrence.

Caffeine

Caffeine consumption is another area where the truth seems to conflict with the common myth. It's often thought that too much coffee can either cause an ulcer or make the symptoms worse. But this doesn't seem to be the case.

It's true that coffee stimulates the secretion of gastric acid. This is true whether the coffee is caffeinated or decaffeinated. But there is no evidence that drinking coffee or lots of caffeinated drinks, such as colas, will cause an ulcer.

However, it appears that if you previously drank a lot of coffee earlier in life you could be more at risk of developing a duodenal ulcer later on. One study of the drinking habits of university students found that consumption of coffee and cola drinks tended to be associated with an increased frequency of ulcer disease later in life.[4] Interestingly, having a high milk intake seemed to be associated with protection from ulcers. However, as yet a strong direct association between caffeine and ulcers cannot be confirmed.

Alcohol Intake

Again, there have been a lot of suggestions that too much alcohol can lead to peptic ulcers. It used to be thought that alcohol stimulated gastrin release and acid secretion. Studies have failed to confirm this.[5,6] So again, there is no clear evidence that alcohol causes or exacerbates (makes worse) peptic ulcers.

That fact is that alcohol drinkers, including both moderate and heavy drinkers, do not have an increased incidence of peptic ulcers. The only exception is people with alcoholic cirrhosis of the liver, who do have an increased incidence of duodenal ulcers. However, this appears to be related to the damage to the liver rather than directly to the alcohol intake itself.

Stress

For a long time it was believed that there was an 'ulcer personality'. The classic stereotype was the harried executive who is under a lot of pressure, eats on the run and drinks his lunch. So far, there is no evidence to support this belief.

It was thought that being under a lot of stress would increase the amount of acid secretion and pepsin. And, although changes in the gastric mucosa and increased secretion do occur when you're under pressure, there is no evidence that stressful life events cause or exacerbate peptic ulcers.

However, stress may play a role in making ulcers worse once they have developed. So, reducing stress may improve healing and help prevent a recurrence (*see Chapter 9 for stress-reducing techniques*).

There are special types of ulcers, called stress ulcers, that do seem to occur when a person is under extreme physical stress, for instance after suffering severe burns or wounds. This can make patients temporarily more vulnerable to developing gastric ulcers. However, these ulcers are different from true peptic ones, and they are treated differently.

Medications

Certain medications and drugs have long been thought to be a causative agent in the development of peptic ulcers. Study after study seems to bear this out. The most common medications thought to contribute to the development of ulcers are aspirin and other non-steroidal anti-inflammatory drugs (NSAIDs), and corticosteroids.

ASPIRIN

People who use aspirin regularly – four or more days a week for three or more months – have an increased risk of getting a gastric ulcer. This is more true in women than in men. Before you panic, it's important to realize that the occasional use of aspirin has no effect on your risk of developing an ulcer.

Many people who regularly take aspirin develop an ulcer, most commonly a 'silent' one with no obvious problems or symptoms. They are also more at risk of developing ulcer complications such as bleeding or perforation, because aspirin can lead to bleeding in the upper gastrointestinal tract.

Why aspirin should have this effect is clear: taking aspirin regularly prevents the formation of the protective prostaglandins. It also damages the gastric mucosa (stomach lining). These two effects can lead to peptic ulcer formation and can also cause existing ulcers to bleed.

NSAIDS

Many elderly people take non-steroidal anti-inflammatory drugs (NSAIDs) on a regular basis to help relieve the pain of chronic conditions such as rheumatoid arthritis and osteoarthritis. NSAIDs are very effective at reducing inflammation, and therefore swelling and pain.

But, as a result, there has been an increase in the number of these people developing ulcer disease. It's estimated that somewhere between 15 and 30 per cent of chronic NSAID users will develop a peptic ulcer at some time in their lives. There is also a higher proportion of people taking NSAIDs who need admission to hospital because of intestinal bleeding or perforation. It's estimated that in the UK, the risk of elderly people developing a bleeding gastric or duodenal ulcer is increased two to four times over the normal rate for people of the same age group who are not taking NSAIDs. This may be related to NSAID intake.

It is thought that the mechanism by which NSAIDs cause ulcers is similar to that for aspirin. NSAIDs, just like aspirin, damage the stomach lining and inhibit the production of the protective prostaglandins.

CORTICOSTEROIDS

This category of drugs has been looked at extensively to see if there is any link between taking them and an increase in the risk of developing an ulcer. Most of the studies concluded that there is no significant risk, unless you are taking fairly high doses of the medication.

It's likely that high or prolonged doses of corticosteroids may increase your risk of developing an ulcer, or can make an existing ulcer worse. And the possibility remains that even moderate doses of corticosteroids may be implicated in causing peptic ulcers.

Acid Output

Gastroenterologists (specialists in digestive tract illnesses) have special tests and investigations which can measure the amount of acid you produce. Initially it was suspected that people who develop ulcers secrete more acid, and that this contributed to their condition.

It is now generally accepted that, as a group, people with duodenal ulcers do secrete more acid than people without ulcers. It's thought this is because they have more parietal cells (the special cells that control acid secretion) in the stomach lining. People with duodenal ulcers also produce more acid during the night than normal.

Whether or not this extra acid contributes to their ulcer is not known. Some studies have found that about 70 to 80 per cent of people with duodenal ulcers who are taking medication will find that their ulcer heals normally, even though they continue to secrete more acid. So it may be that other factors are more important in the development of their disease than the fact that they secrete more acid.

In people with gastric ulcers the picture is less clear. Most patients with gastric ulcers produce normal amounts of acid. In fact, some patients with gastric ulcers have even a lower acid output than normal. So in their case acid-production may be even less significant when considering factors that trigger ulcers.

Genetic Factors

It's been known for almost 50 years that a tendency to peptic ulcers may run in families. Siblings of people with peptic ulcers are about 2.5 times more likely to develop them. It's also known that, within families, one type of ulcer tends to prevail. If your brother is prone to duodenal ulcers, it's more likely that, if you get an ulcer, it will be a duodenal ulcer rather than a stomach ulcer.

Initially it was considered that peptic ulcers might be inherited — just like some cancers or heart disease. With the discovery of *Helicobacter pylori*, it's now thought that cross-infection with the bug makes family members more likely to develop the same condition.

Nor is it clear whether there are racial patterns to peptic ulcer disease. Epidemiological studies have shown that some races or ethnic groups are more likely to develop ulcers than others. But it is difficult for scientists to determine exactly why this should be. It could be that different races have a different inherited susceptibility to ulcers, or it could be related to the fact that they are exposed to different environmental factors, such as diet. And it could also be that *Helicobacter pylori* affects certain races of people and not others, making them more likely to get infected.

It is known that your blood group will definitely make a difference in your risk of developing a duodenal ulcer. People of blood group O are about 25 per cent more likely to develop duodenal ulcers. It's thought that these people have more parietal cells than normal. These are the cells that are responsible for the secretion of hydrochloric acid from the stomach.

In about 80 per cent of the population (regardless of their blood group) a special substance called AB antigen is secreted in the saliva and other gastric juices. This substance appears to have a protective effect, strengthening the barrier of the stomach lining from pepsin and acid. So people who do not secrete this special antigen (non-secretors) have been found to be about 30 per cent more susceptible to developing duodenal ulcers.

The pattern in gastric ulcers is less clear. Some data suggests a similar picture to that seen in cases of duodenal ulcer. Other studies have indicated that gastric ulcers are slightly more common in people with blood group A.

Why your blood group makes a difference isn't exactly clear. So far there has been no proven correlation between acid or pepsin secretion and blood group status. However, one thought is that blood group proteins, called antigens, are expressed or marked on stomach cells. And this may be how *H. pylori* can stick to the stomach cells – it literally attaches itself to these sticky proteins on the cells of the stomach lining. And it seems to stick more to some blood group proteins than others.

Links with Other Diseases

Peptic ulcers can occur in conjunction with other conditions. One rare condition, called Zollinger-Ellison syndrome, causes exorbitant amounts of acid to be produced in the stomach. People with Zollinger-Ellison syndrome are especially prone to both duodenal and gastric ulcers. This is because they have one or several tumours, usually in the pancreas, which secrete the hormone gastrin. And gastrin stimulates the stomach to produce large quantities of acid.

Many people do not realize they have Zollinger-Ellison syndrome until they are treated for peptic ulcers. But when the condition is discovered and the tumours removed, you cure the disease. Anti-ulcer medication can also be given to heal the ulcers.

Duodenal ulcers may occur in conjunction with other conditions, including cystic fibrosis and Crohn's disease. Many other illnesses have been claimed to increase your risk of developing chronic peptic ulcer, including chronic kidney disease and hyperparathyroidism. Low blood pressure also seems to increase your risk of developing peptic ulcers, although why this should be isn't known.

The Myths and the Facts

- Cigarette smokers are about twice as likely to have ulcers than non-smokers.
- Alcohol seems to have no effect on the development of peptic ulcers.
- High-fibre diets seem to protect against the occurrence of duodenal ulcers. They may also protect against the reoccurrence of a duodenal ulcer.
- People who regularly take aspirin or NSAIDs are at increased risk of developing a gastric ulcer. This is more true for women than for men.
- Caffeine seems to have no immediate effect on the development of an ulcer. Drinking large amounts of coffee earlier in life may predispose a person to an ulcer later in life.
- There is no 'ulcer personality'. Stress does not cause or lead to an ulcer.

5

THE FIRST STEPS TO HELP

For most people who suffer from symptoms they suspect are due to an ulcer, the first step should be a visit to their general practitioner. Many of you may have tried over-the-counter remedies such as antacids instead of making an appointment with the doctor. It may be that you don't want to bother your doctor, or you find that the treatments from the chemist do help in the short term.

But the treatments you can buy without a prescription, including antacids and certain formulations of H_2 antagonists, are not really designed to treat peptic ulcer disease. They do help with symptoms such as heartburn and indigestion, but will not heal an ulcer quickly or keep it healed in the long term.

If you've been putting off seeing your doctor about your symptoms, make an appointment now. It is the only way you'll be able to get a proper diagnosis and treatment for your condition.

As yet there are no official guidelines on the 'correct' way of diagnosing and treating peptic ulcer disease. Different doctors, depending on their background and beliefs, as well as whether they belong to fund-holding or non-fund-holding practices, will treat ulcer patients in different ways. What sort of health facilities are available in your area also plays a part in the type of treatment you receive.

Some doctors may test you for *Helicobacter pylori* infection, others will prescribe a course of medication and wait to see if the symptoms clear up. If it is easy to refer you for endoscopy – a diagnostic technique which involves inserting a tiny telescope into the stomach to look for an ulcer – you may be sent for this. There are just no hard and fast rules.

What type of investigations you have will also depend on a number of factors, including your age. People over 45 are more at risk of stomach cancer, so if you show up complaining about pain and are younger than 45, your doctor may assume it's an ulcer rather than anything more sinister. If you are over this age, your doctor may send you for investigation before prescribing treatment. This is to exclude the possibility of your symptoms being due to gastric cancer. It is likely that treatment will be withheld until the results of the investigations are known.

It's important to keep all this in mind when discussing your condition with your GP. Don't be alarmed if your doctor recommends a course of treatment that is different from that prescribed for a friend or relative with similar symptoms. It does not mean the treatment is incorrect – just that your doctor has many appropriate options, and is choosing the one most suitable for you.

Table overleaf reproduced by kind permission of Medical Imprint

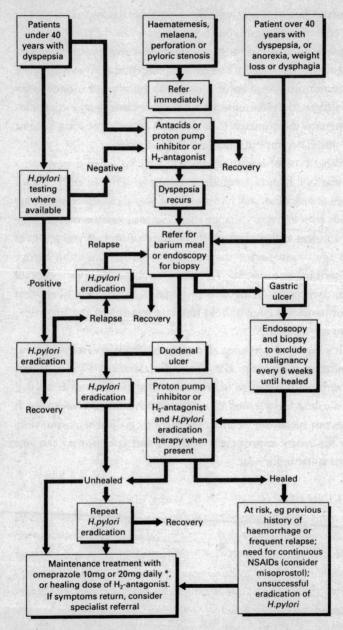

* *Lansoprazole is not licensed for this indication*

Seeing the Doctor

Probably one of the more common reasons for a visit to the doctor is dyspepsia, or indigestion. Although this is a primary symptom of ulcer disease, there are a number of other causes and not all of them are ulcer-related. For instance, indigestion is a symptom of gallstones as well as inflammation of the oesophagus. So your doctor will want to determine the primary – or main – cause of your symptoms.

All doctors will want to take a full medical history. Yours will probably ask very detailed questions about your symptoms. For instance, he or she will want to know how long you have had your symptoms, exactly what they are, how often they occur, and how severe they are.

Your GP will also ask you about your diet and lifestyle. Do you smoke cigarettes, do you eat a lot of fatty foods, do you drink alcohol? The answers to these and other specific questions will provide clues as to the cause of your pain.

The doctor may even ask detailed questions about the pain. Can you pinpoint where it hurts? What time of the day does it occur most often? Do you wake up at night in pain? How long do the attacks last, and do you find that eating makes the pain better or worse?

All of these questions help the doctor build up a true picture of your condition.

TAKING NOTES

All of us get nervous when we go to the doctor. And though you may be in agony at the time of an ulcer attack, it is often difficult to remember afterwards the exact nature of your pain, how severe it was and when it occurred. By the time you get to the doctor, your ulcer attack may seem like a distant memory.

For this reason it is a good idea to make a note of your symptoms as they occur. If possible, before your appointment try to keep a diary and write down the following:

- the time and date of your ulcer attacks
- what foods or drinks you had beforehand
- any medications you are taking (don't forget to include simple over-the-counter ones like painkillers, vitamins or cold remedies)
- whether or not certain foods or drinks seem to help relieve the pain
- how long the attacks last
- whether attacks are worse at night, or cause you to wake up in the night in pain
- any symptoms such as nausea, vomiting, or blood in the stools
- how long you have had the symptoms – weeks, months, years?
- any over-the-counter medications you have been taking for the pain, and whether these have helped.

It is possible that your doctor will also want to perform a physical examination, paying pretty close attention to your abdomen. He or she may ask if you can point to the area in which the pain seems to be located. Many ulcer patients find they can be very specific – they often point to almost the exact location of the ulcer, using their fingertip. However, the pain of ulcers can spread all around your abdomen and your back. This may make it difficult for you to be exact, so don't be too concerned if your answer is a more general one.

Getting Treatment

In most cases peptic ulcer disease can initially be treated by your GP. If the symptoms are extremely severe, or if your doctor suspects you may have complications, you may be referred to a gastroenterologist at the local hospital.

It could be that your age makes a difference. Because of the risk of stomach cancer, your GP may prefer you to be investigated by a specialist and you may be cared for thereafter by that specialist.

If you are young and this is the first sign of peptic ulcer disease, it's highly likely your GP will give you a prescription for an ulcer-healing drug, such as an H_2 antagonist, without any further investigation. In most cases the prescription will be for a month's treatment. The doctor will then ask you to come back after that time to reassess your condition.

After that time, in about a quarter of patients the ulcer does seem to heal. If this is true in your case, you will need no further treatment unless you suffer a recurrence.

However, for the majority of patients the symptoms do not clear up, or do not clear sufficiently. It's estimated that, without eradication therapy to eliminate *Helicobacter pylori*, almost 80 per cent of patients will have a recurrence of their ulcer, often within months of initially successful treatment and certainly within the first year after treatment.

If this is the case with you, or if this is not the first time you have seen your doctor about your symptoms, you probably will then be referred for some type of upper gastrointestinal tract investigation, such as a barium meal or endoscopy. (*For more information, see Chapter 6*). Once the results of these investigations are known, your doctor can then tailor the treatment more effectively for your needs.

Testing for *Helicobacter pylori*

Although the discovery of *H. pylori* and its role in ulcer disease
has drastically changed attitudes, it is highly unlikely you will
be treated for *H. pylori* infection until you have first been tested to confirm the presence of the bacteria.

As yet there are no guidelines in the UK on testing for *H.
pylori*. In the United States, where ulcer disease is also a huge
problem, the National Institutes of Health (NIH) issued a consensus statement in 1994. They have come to the conclusion
that ulcer patients who are known to be infected with *H. pylori*
should be treated with antibiotics in addition to anti-secretory
drugs, whether it's the first time a patient has seen the doctor
about the illness or if he or she is suffering a recurrence.

As a result, patients in the US may be more likely to be tested to see if they are infected with *H. pylori*. However, in the
UK this is not yet the case.

If you have an endoscopy, in almost all cases they will take a
biopsy (tissue sample) from the stomach area and test in the
laboratory for *H. pylori*.

Not all patients with peptic ulcer symptoms will have an
endoscopy. But even patients who are not endoscoped can be
tested, too. One way to do this is with blood tests.

Unfortunately, these tests are not generally covered by the
National Health Service. If your GP's practice is a fund-holding one, these tests can come out of the practice budget. If
your practice is non-fund-holding, and remember this is still
true of the majority, you will either have to go to hospital to
have the test, or be willing to pay the cost – around £14 –
yourself. If you do decide to pay yourself, you get a private
prescription for the test, pick it up at the pharmacy and take
the test back to the doctor's. This eliminates the need for a
hospital appointment and may help speed up your treatment.

If you have the test performed in hospital, the results will be sent back to your GP, who will discuss the results with you at a later appointment.

There are also breath tests that can be used to detect *H. pylori*. These tests measure the amount of carbon dioxide in exhaled breath. You may be given a substance called urea with carbon to drink. Bacteria, such as *H. pylori*, break down this urea and the carbon is absorbed into the bloodstream and lungs and exhaled when you breathe. By then testing your breath, doctors can measure the carbon and determine whether *H. pylori* is present or absent. These urea breath tests are at least 90 per cent accurate for diagnosing the bacteria. As yet this type of test is not widely available or used, but hopefully this should soon change.

Case Study – Seeing the Doctor

I'd been having some problems for almost 18 months before I finally went to see my family doctor. It turned into a real bad problem. At first I didn't consider it too serious. I just thought I had an ulcer, which is pretty common. So I started taking loads of remedies you can buy over the counter at the pharmacy to help keep things under control.

At first the tablets and liquids seemed to help and the discomfort would disappear, at least for quite a while. But after a while I found they weren't as effective as they were initially. I'd take some antacid or something similar, and it would help for just a brief time, a few minutes or half an hour. Then the pain would start to come back. I just couldn't keep it under control. I found that because I felt so terrible all the time, I was having real trouble eating. I felt as if I couldn't keep anything down, or was worried that whatever I ate would upset my stomach. I started losing weight, and felt tired all the time and didn't have any energy.

Finally I couldn't take it anymore. I remember one night being out with my wife and friends and it was so uncomfortable I just had to go home and lie down. That was the final straw for me. Even my wife told me she was going to make an appointment for me if I wouldn't.

When I explained my symptoms, the doctor suspected I had an ulcer, which is what I imagined my problem to be. He prescribed some tablets, which I took morning and evening. They seemed to do the trick, and I continued taking them for about four weeks. They made such a difference. The pain eased up in less than a week, and they worked much better than anything I'd bought from the pharmacies.

But at the same time I decided I didn't want to take anything long term, and made some changes to my diet. I stopped eating a lot of junk foods, and tried to include healthier foods like fruit and vegetables. So far I haven't had any more problems. But if the ulcer does come back, I won't put off seeing the doctor like before. I know that there's little I can do myself, and will get help right away to avoid going through that agony again.

CHRIS, 29

6

DIAGNOSING AN ULCER

Once you have seen your GP and discussed your symptoms and condition, he or she will probably have a very good idea of whether or not the cause of your problems is an ulcer. But because ulcers are an internal condition which cannot be seen, your doctor cannot be absolutely sure unless you have had some type of investigation. This is done by specialists in hospital, and only then can the diagnosis be truly confirmed.

Diagnosing an ulcer is not a complicated process, and the investigations available will determine if you do have an ulcer, how large it is, and exactly where in the stomach or duodenum it is located.

In some cases you may have already had some form of prescribed treatment, such as H_2 antagonists, before going on for further investigation. The need for investigation usually arises because the treatment has failed to eliminate your symptoms, or because treatment was initially successful but you have had a recurrence of your symptoms. In other cases your doctor may want to confirm the diagnosis before starting treatment. In any case, the procedures are the same.

The Tests Available

There are two types of test or investigation for peptic ulcers: barium meal X-rays and endoscopy. The type of investigation you have will depend on your GP, your condition, and the facilities available in your area, which will also determine the waiting time.

In many areas around the UK, barium meals can often be performed more quickly – that is, there will be a shorter wait for an appointment – than endoscopy. But the National Health Service has recently streamlined the waiting process for endoscopy with what is called 'open access' endoscopy.

Contrary to what it sounds like, this is not a different procedure. What this relates to is the way in which you are referred for testing. In the past this was a two-step procedure. Your GP or family doctor would first have to send to you a gastroenterologist at the local hospital. It would then be the gastroenterologist who sent you on for endoscopy, usually at the same hospital.

But open access endoscopy has changed all of this. If the facilities are available in your area, your doctor can now refer you directly for testing, in much the same way you would be referred for a chest X-ray, and indeed a barium meal, which do not require a visit to a specialist first.

BARIUM MEALS

In Britain, barium meals are still performed more frequently than endoscopy for diagnosing ulcer disease. However, this picture is changing and barium X-rays are no longer used as widely as before. In the future, as more endoscopy centres are opened, it is likely that the first line of investigation will be endoscopy.

Although a barium meal is less expensive than endoscopy,

less invasive and there is usually a shorter waiting time at hospital centres, it has some major drawbacks as a diagnostic tool.

First, barium meals are less accurate than endoscopy. In about 30 per cent of cases, they provide an incorrect diagnosis. They do not provide as much information as endoscopy. They are not particularly effective in picking up very small ulcers, and they are not especially good at pinpointing the exact size and depth of an ulcer. Nor can they detect the presence of *Helicobacter pylori*. In spite of these drawbacks, barium meals are still effective at diagnosing a peptic ulcer.

How It Is Done

Barium sulphate is a metallic salt that is visible on X-ray pictures. It is used in a number of investigative procedures to show up areas of the digestive tract that need to be checked out.

Because barium cannot be taken in its raw form, the powdered barium sulphate is made up into a mixture, or 'meal', and swallowed. This helps coat the lining of the stomach and duodenum, and enables it to be seen clearly on an X-ray picture. The barium coats the craters or holes of an ulcer as well, and shows them as white spots on the X-rays. These spots are picked up by the radiologist (a doctor specially trained in interpreting X-ray images).

The procedure is done on an out-patient basis in the radiology department of a hospital. It is painless and no anaesthetic is needed. It is very safe, though it can be uncomfortable for some patients.

Before you go in for a barium meal you will be given a list of instructions about what to do. Depending on the time you are having the barium meal, you will be asked not to eat or drink anything for at least six to nine hours beforehand. This helps ensure that there is no food left in the digestive tract when the X-ray is taken.

Once you are ready for your barium meal, it will be mixed up and you will be given the barium in the form of a drink. Usually the powdered barium will be mixed with a flavoured liquid. The mixture can be thick and chalky, although barium meals tend to be less liquid in texture than barium swallows, which are used for other diagnostic procedures of the upper gastrointestinal tract. You may find that you need to drink quite a lot of the mixture, and may also need to drink it in stages.

You may also be asked to drink carbonated water along with the barium, or you may be asked to take a special tablet or small granules which will create carbon dioxide in your stomach. This helps to distend, or bloat, the stomach and the duodenum. This helps to provide a better image and improve the accuracy of the X-rays.

The radiologist will wait a certain amount of time (usually around 5 to 10 minutes) before taking the first pictures, to give the barium time to reach the relevant part of your digestive tract. You will be asked both to stand for X-rays and also to lie on the table in various positions while the X-rays are taken. This is so the radiologist can get pictures of your stomach or duodenum from various angles, to ensure that no part is overlooked.

The number of X-rays you have will depend on the type of ulcer suspected, and also on the radiologist. However, the entire procedure from the start of taking X-rays lasts only about 10 to 15 minutes.

After the Barium Meal

Because you have ingested barium sulphate, you may find that this causes you to become constipated. Doctors are aware of this problem and will usually give you some laxatives or a prescription to take away with you. You may be advised to eat a fibre-rich diet to help avoid constipation, and to drink plenty of fluid to help get rid of the remaining barium. This can take up to four days, depending on your bowel habits. You may also find your stools become a bit white in colour afterwards. This is nothing to worry about.

The radiologist will interpret your X-rays. Although the results of your barium meal may be known immediately, he or she may not tell you straight away what has been found. Instead, a full report of the findings, and possibly the X-rays or copies of the X-ray pictures, will be sent to your GP or specialist. You will then be called back to see your doctor or specialist, who will discuss the results with you and decide on treatment.

ENDOSCOPY

The advent and development of endoscopy has made it the first choice in diagnosing peptic ulcers.

Endoscopy is a method of looking directly at various internal areas of the body. It is used for both diagnosis and, sometimes, treatment.

When endoscopy is used for investigating the stomach and intestine, you may hear the procedure referred to as 'gastroscopy'. Other endoscopic procedures are used for different areas of the body. For example, laparoscopy refers to investigation of the abdomen, while arthroscopy is the term used for endoscopy of the joints.

Many of the endoscopes used for these different procedures are fundamentally the same. An endoscope, which is similar to a long tube or telescope, usually has fibre optics on one end. This allows light to be bent along flexible tubes which the doctor can 'steer' to get the best look.

The newer generation of endoscopes don't use fibre optics. Instead, they have a tiny video chip on the end of the scope.

This chip sends signals back to the monitor, where they are turned into images of the inside of your stomach or duodenum which can be viewed by the specialist. Endoscopes are tiny, only about 1 cm (less than half an inch) in diameter, even though they also contain viewing and illumination equipment.

The controls at the viewing end allow the tip of the steerable endoscope to be turned in any direction. This allows the doctor to view the stomach and the duodenum, and also helps ensure that he or she can check out every part of these areas, without missing any.

The endoscope can be used to obtain colour photographs or video recordings of the area. In addition, tiny instruments can be attached to the endoscope. This allows the specialist to remove a tiny sample of tissue (perform a biopsy) to be examined later.

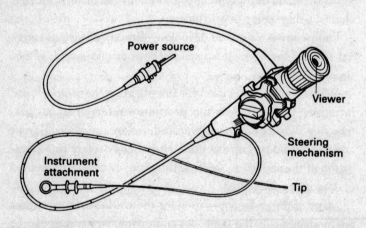

An Endoscope

How It Is Done

As with barium meals, endoscopy is performed on an out-patient basis at the hospital. Again, you will be asked to abstain from eating or drinking anything for about six to eight hours before the procedure.

Because endoscopy can cause mild discomfort (though it is not painful), the back of your mouth and throat will usually be sprayed with a local anaesthetic. This helps to numb the area and reduce any discomfort. It also helps to suppress your gagging and coughing reflexes, which normally occur when any object touches the back of your throat. You may also be given a mild sedative, usually an intravenous dose of a drug such as diazepam, beforehand to help relax you during the procedure. Some endoscopists combine this with a drug that helps relax the smooth muscles of the oesophagus and stomach.

You will be asked to lie on your left side. A protective device or mouthpiece is usually placed between your teeth to stop you biting the endoscope. The tip of the endoscope is then introduced through the mouthpiece, and you'll be encouraged to swallow. This helps the endoscope to go down your throat.

Once the tip of the endoscope is in position, air may be blown in to inflate the stomach. This distension of the stomach aids the inspection of the area. It may cause some minor discomfort, but it is not usually painful.

The endoscope is then passed through the throat into the stomach and the duodenum. You may feel the tip of the instrument rubbing against the internal stomach wall, especially as it will be rotated and turned in a number of directions to get a full picture of your upper digestive tract.

During the examination the images will appear on a monitor near the endoscopist. This allows him or her to see the exact state of your stomach and duodenum. In many cases the doctor can actually take colour photographs or images of the area. Because the doctor is viewing the inside of your stomach or duodenum, he or she can see precisely any signs of an ulcer, exactly where it is, how big it is and how deep it is. The entire examination takes only about 20 minutes.

Case Study – Endoscopy

I've suffered from a duodenal ulcer since I was in my twenties. I took different tablets for years, including Tagamet and Zantac. I'd take them every night, and they usually worked fairly well. But if I ate too much, or drank red wine or had lots of rich, creamy foods, I knew I was in for some trouble the next day.

I'd always put off having an endoscopy because I thought it would be uncomfortable. I work in a local hospital as an administrator, and knew a little bit about the procedure. I thought it would be painful, and I didn't like the idea of them putting a tube down my throat.

Finally my doctor convinced me that I really should have one. My ulcer was acting up even with me taking my tablets, and he wanted to make sure there was nothing more serious going on. So I finally made an appointment and went in for an endoscopy.

I have to admit I was nervous about it, but the doctor and nurses were very kind and very calming. They explained everything to me beforehand, so I knew exactly what to expect. I had an injection in my arm of a sedative to keep me calm, and then they asked me to open my mouth wide. They also sprayed my throat with a local anaesthetic. And before you could say nowt, the tube was down my throat.

I thought it would be terribly uncomfortable, but it wasn't. I could feel a funny sensation when they turned the tube this way and that. But it didn't take long. It seemed that within seconds it was over, though I know it took about 20 minutes or so.

My husband was waiting to fetch me home, and I felt fine afterwards, although my throat was a little sore. It wasn't at all what I expected, and I'm sorry it took me so long to have one. The results showed that I was infected with Helicobacter pylori, and so I had a course of eradication therapy to eliminate the bacteria. This helped to clear my ulcer completely.

JUDITH, 53

Having a Biopsy

By attaching tiny instruments to the tip of the endoscope, the doctor can also take a sample of tissue for biopsy. This tissue sample is then sent off to the laboratory and checked for any signs of malignancy, such as gastric cancer, or the presence of *Helicobacter pylori*.

If your doctor suspects you have a stomach ulcer, a biopsy is usually performed. This is because stomach ulcers can sometimes be malignant, or cancerous. However, if you have a duodenal ulcer, a biopsy may not be performed, because duodenal ulcers are never malignant.

After the Endoscopy

After endoscopy you may notice that you have a slightly sore throat. In the past some patients found that they experienced a little bleeding in their stools, which resulted from the friction of the instruments against the lining of the throat and stomach. This was fairly rare, and the newer endoscopes usually prevent this from occurring.

If you have had a spray anaesthetic applied to your throat, you should not eat or drink anything for about an hour after the endoscopy because your mouth and back of your throat may still be numb. If you have had a mild sedative, you will probably be advised not to drive or operate heavy machinery for 24 hours afterwards. The hospital will probably have asked you to make arrangements for collection from the hospital.

Once you have had an endoscopy, after about a week or so the report will be posted or faxed back to your GP or specialist. It will include the results of any biopsy that was performed, and will indicate whether there were any signs of either cancer or. *Helicobacter pylori* infection.

The report will usually tell your doctor what type of ulcer you have, where it is located, and an estimation of its size and severity. In some cases a photograph of the ulcer will be included. You will be asked to go back to your doctor to discuss the results and decide on the best course of treatment for you.

Testing for *Helicobacter Pylori*

There are a number of different investigations which can be used to detect the presence of the bacterium *Helicobacter pylori*. If you are having endoscopy, a biopsy (tissue sample) will be sent to the laboratory for examination. Blood or serum tests can also be used to detect the presence of *H. pylori*.

However, these tests can really only tell whether or not you have been infected with *H. pylori* at some time – they cannot actually confirm that the infection is still active. This is because the tests look for antibodies to *H. pylori* in the blood. These are the chemicals produced by your body when fighting an infection. *H. pylori* antibodies can stay in your system for quite a long time after the infection has been eradicated. For this reason, blood tests are more useful if administered *before* any ulcer treatment, to see if eradication therapy would be useful. They are not useful for checking whether eradication therapy has been successful, because you may still have antibodies in your system even though the bug itself is no longer present.

A simpler test is being developed, using saliva rather than blood, but this is not yet commercially available. When it does come onto the market it is likely that many GPs will take the opportunity of carrying out the test in their own practice rather than referring you to hospital. However, a test of this kind will be less accurate than one that goes to a laboratory for analysis.

The urea breath tests mentioned earlier are also effective, though not yet widely available around the UK.

7

TREATING AN ULCER

In the past, ulcers were thought to be a result of too much stress, a rich diet and high living – the 'hurry, worry and curry' syndrome. As a result, some treatments were used that may sound very strange to us today.

One well-known treatment used around the time of the First World War was called the Sippy Diet. It was named after the American Bertram Sippy, and involved giving people with peptic ulcers plenty of milk and cream. This high-fat, high-cholesterol regime usually started with hourly feedings of milk and cream, then added eggs, custards and puréed foods. Sippy thought that the crucial element in treating ulcers was continuous control of gastric acid. If there was no acid, there was no ulcer. And dairy foods were thought to suppress the production of stomach acid, reducing the incidence of new ulcers and speeding the healing of existing ones.

Today, most gastroenterologists believe that, when it comes to ulcers, what you eat is irrelevant. And the Sippy diet is clearly obsolete.

Bed rest was another former treatment for ulcers. By keeping activity (and therefore, it was believed, stress) to a minimum, it was thought that ulcers would heal better.

As experts learned more and more about the causes of ulcers, treatment recommendations changed. As mentioned, the discovery of the role that *Helicobacter pylori* plays in the development of ulcer disease has again dramatically altered the way ulcers are treated.

Guidelines for Treatment

The recent consensus statement from the National Institutes of Health (NIH) in the US describes *Helicobacter pylori* as having a profound effect on the current thinking on peptic ulcer disease. The authors of this statement recommend that ulcer patients with *H. pylori* should be treated with antibiotics in addition to drugs which reduce the secretion of acid, whether this is the first time the patients present to their doctor with symptoms or if they are suffering a relapse or recurrence.

As yet, no firm guidelines have been established in Britain by the Department of Health or organizations such as the British Society of Gastroenterology (BSG), although it is likely that the BSG will be providing recommendations of care for their members in the very near future.

Keeping this in mind, the treatment you receive will depend on a number of different factors. These can include your doctor and his or her knowledge about ulcers, the hospital you are being treated at, and the area in which you live. Even the cost of medication will influence your treatment, as some forms are much more expensive (though not necessarily more effective) than others and your doctor may choose to prescribe a less expensive medication initially.

Once your doctor has determined you have a peptic ulcer, and this may be from your history and symptoms or from the results of investigations such as endoscopy, you will probably initially be started on one of the proven ulcer medications. You may also be given some form of eradication therapy for *Heli-cobacter pylori*, even if you have not actually been tested for the presence of the bacterium.

What's Available

There are a number of medicines used to heal and prevent the recurrence of peptic ulcers. In general, the drugs used to treat peptic ulcer disease work in four different ways:

1 Antacids neutralize or buffer the effects of stomach acid.
2 Both H_2 antagonists and proton pump inhibitors inhibit the secretion of gastric acid.
3 Drugs such as sucralfate improve the defence mechanisms of the stomach's mucosal lining.
4 Antibiotics eradicate the bacterium *Helicobacter pylori*.

Some of the drugs have more than one effect, and you may find that you are given a prescription for a combination of drugs rather than just one. You may also find that one drug does not effectively eliminate your symptoms and heal your ulcer. If so, your doctor may try another similar medication to see if it suits you better. In many cases it is a matter of trial and error. This is very common with ulcers, so do not be concerned if your initial course of treatment is unsuccessful. The second is likely to be.

Antacids

Antacids have been the mainstay of ulcer treatment for many years. The formal use of antacids is said to have begun in 1856, when William Brinton, a Londoner, first used bicarbonate of potash and also bismuth to treat gastric ulcers (gastric ulcers themselves had first been described in Paris in 1835, by Jean Cruveilhier).

In the US the popularity of antacids took off with the work of Bertram Sippy in 1915. In the following 50 years, antacids were widely used; their popularity grew further when in 1952 it was demonstrated that neutralizing the acidic contents of the stomach helped relieve pain in patients with peptic ulcers.

Until the British discovery of H_2 antagonists in the mid-1970s, antacids were the principal form of treatment. With the development of more effective ulcer drugs, the use of antacids has fallen by the wayside. They can be effective in reducing a lot of the symptoms, but they no longer have a major role to play in healing ulcers. Because so many people buy them from pharmacies as a first line of treatment when they begin to get symptoms, however, it is important to know a bit about how they work and what effects they have.

HOW THEY WORK

Antacids work by neutralizing the stomach acids that have already been secreted into the stomach and duodenum. They do not stop acid from being secreted in the first place. This is why antacids only provide temporary relief from pain.

There are a number of different compounds used as antacids, and they usually come in liquid, tablet or gel form. The liquids work more quickly than the tablets, so you may find these more useful if you require speedy relief.

Antacids in tablet form are often considered more convenient from the patient's point of view. And, as better tablet formulations become available, they may soon rival the liquids for effectiveness. Because the relief all antacids provide is only temporary, lasting a few hours or slightly longer, you will need to take them regularly throughout the day for them to be of any use.

A number of antacids are available over the counter. These will vary tremendously in their ability to relieve the burning pain of excess acid. Eventually you may find that they provide little or no relief, and you will need to progress to a stronger formulation or some other type of drug.

The most common antacids are the ones that contain either calcium aluminium, or magnesium. The different compounds will also have different side-effects (*see below*).

For a long time bicarbonate of soda was the antacid most frequently taken by ulcer sufferers. Bicarbonate of soda is absorbed into the body and goes on to disturb the balance of acid in the blood and tissues. Newer antacids, called non-absorbable antacids, are not absorbed into the bloodstream in this way.

SIDE-EFFECTS

Different antacids will have different side-effects, depending on their constituents. It's fairly well accepted that high doses of certain antacids, particularly ones that contain magnesium, can cause diarrhoea. One study from 1977 published in the *New England Journal of Medicine* found that around 30 per cent of patients taking high doses of antacids developed this problem.[1]

Antacids that contain aluminium lead to the opposite problem – that is, they are known to cause constipation. For this reason some antacids are combined with agents that help prevent constipation by loosening the stool.

Other antacids may contain high levels of sodium, so they are not usually given to patients with hypertension (high blood pressure) or those on a low-salt diet.

Another common problem with antacids is that they can interfere with the absorption of other medications you may be taking, such as some antibiotics. It is very important, therefore, that if you are thinking of taking antacids you let your doctor or pharmacist know if you are on any other medication already.

HOW EFFECTIVE ARE THEY?

It was initially thought that antacids could only be used to relieve the pain of peptic ulcers, and that even then they could not provide particularly effective or long-term relief.

Clinical trials have shown that they *are* in fact effective at speeding up the healing of ulcers. However, they must be given in fairly high doses, and be taken reasonably frequently, to have this healing effect. It also appears that antacids are better at healing duodenal ulcers than stomach ulcers.

With the development of better anti-ulcer medication, antacids are rarely used on their own these days. In some cases they may be given along with other ulcer-healing drugs, or as part of eradication therapy for *Helicobacter pylori*.

H$_2$ Antagonists

In the mid 1970s a new class of drugs, called H$_2$ antagonists, created a revolution in the treatment of ulcer disease.

HOW THEY WORK

For many years it's been known that histamine, a chemical released by special cells in the body (called mast cells) is a powerful stimulant of gastric acid secretion. However, this stimulating effect is not blocked, nor prevented, by conventional antihistamines you might take for, say, allergy symptoms. Noting this, Scottish pharmacologist Sir James Black and his colleagues investigated the function of a second H$_2$ receptor, or histamine 2 receptor, which was found primarily in the gastric mucosa, or lining of the stomach. They were able to demonstrate that the main effect of these H$_2$ receptors in humans is to promote gastric secretion of stomach acids. The H_2 receptors and histamine work like a lock and key. When histamine, the 'key', attaches itself to the H_2 receptors, this opens the 'lock' and allows stomach acids to be released. Sir James Black was awarded a Nobel Prize for his work with H_2 receptors.

As a result of these findings, drugs were developed that block the ability of histamine to 'unlock' the receptors, thereby inhibiting acid secretion. But they do more than just inhibit acid secretion when histamine is present. They also inhibit acid secretion when the vagus nerve is stimulated, and in the presence of food. And by doing so, they enable ulcers to heal fairly quickly. These drugs were given the name H_2 antagonists.

The first potent H_2 antagonist was called metiamide. It is no longer in use; its successor is called cimetidine (trade name Tagamet). A further H_2 antagonist, ranitidine (Zantac) then became extremely popular. More recently famotidine (Pepcid) became available and has proved very useful in healing ulcers. Another H_2 antagonist, nizatidine (Axid) is also available.

HOW EFFECTIVE ARE THEY?

Any number of studies have been carried out to compare the healing rates of the different H_2 antagonists. The results have shown no major differences between them, although pharmaceutical companies would like you to believe that their product is more effective than its competitors. The general consensus is that complete healing rates for any of the H_2 antagonists are around 78 per cent after four weeks and 92 per cent after eight weeks of treatment.

You may have also noticed drugs with similar names, such as Tagamet 100 and Pepcid AC being made available over the counter at pharmacies. These, too, work by blocking the secretion of stomach acid. However, these formulations are generally of a lower dosage than the ones prescribed by a doctor for the treatment of ulcers. These versions are really licensed for use in conditions such as heartburn and dyspepsia (indigestion), not ulcers.

If you have tried them, you may have found initial relief from the symptoms of ulcers, such as pain. But these over-the-counter varieties are not generally strong enough to heal ulcers in a short amount of time, nor to keep them healed in the long term.

CIMETIDINE

You may know cimetidine, the first H_2 antagonist, by its trade name, Tagamet. Tagamet is available in the form of tablet, syrup, injection and infusion. It is effective in reducing the amount of gastric acid secreted, and also reduces pepsin output.

Tagamet is usually taken orally. For most patients with duodenal or gastric ulcers, a single daily dose of 800 milligrams (mg) at bedtime is recommended. You can also split your dose, taking 400 mg at breakfast and another 400 mg at bedtime.

Treatment is usually given initially for four weeks. This might be increased to six weeks for gastric ulcers, and up to eight weeks for ulcers that have been associated with the use of NSAIDs. Most of these ulcers will heal in that time. If healing has not occurred, a second dose may safely be given.

To maintain effective healing, the daily dose should be decreased to 400 mg a day. Again, the most effective way to take this is in one dose before you go to bed. However, splitting the dose into 200 mg in the morning and 200 mg at night has also been shown to be effective.

How Effective Is It?

Years of clinical trials have provided overwhelming evidence that cimetidine is highly effective in healing ulcers in the short term. A number of double-blind controlled trials have been done using cimetidine and placebos. All have confirmed that four to six weeks of treatment with cimetidine helps heal duodenal ulcers.

Prolonging treatment with cimetidine increases the healing rate of duodenal ulcers, by up to as much as 90 per cent after three months. For gastric ulcers the healing rate is about 75 per cent.

Unfortunately, one problem with cimetidine is that the relapse rate is high. Although the initial ulcer is successfully healed, it returns – or recurs – sometime after the course of treatment.

The figures vary from country to country, as cimetidine is used round the world. But about two thirds of patients appear to relapse within the first six months, and a further 15 per cent will have their ulcer back within a year.

Controlled trials have shown that about 15 to 30 per cent of ulcers recur without causing any symptoms. This means that you are unaware that your ulcer has returned. This can be dangerous, because if such silent ulcers go untreated they can lead to complications such as bleeding and perforation.

Even by prolonging treatment there's no difference in the relapse rate. One study looked at whether giving treatment for one, three to six months or a year would help reduce the relapse rate after treatment has been stopped. But the relapse rate appeared to be the same no matter how long the initial course of treatment lasted.

Non-compliance – the patients not following the treatment correctly or consistently – could be one problem. This is a likely possibility if you are on long-term drug therapy.

Side-effects

As with almost any medication, cimetidine can have side-effects. Some of these are related to the drug itself, while others may be related to the effect of blocking the histamine H_2 receptors. Some of the effects are mild, or minor, and will disappear over time or when treatment is stopped. Others may be more serious, and could mean that you need to switch to another drug of the same type or class.

Because cimetidine has been around longer than the other H_2 antagonists, much more is known about its possible side-effects. Drug interaction is probably the most important unwanted effect. This occurs as a result of your altered metabolism when taking cimetidine. Cimetidine can interact with other drugs you may be taking, including the tranquillizer diazepam, the anticoagulant warfarin, and phenytoin, an anti-epilepsy drug. This has to be kept in mind when your doctor prescribes cimetidine for you. Alcohol may counter the beneficial effects of the drug, so you may be advised to avoid alcohol while taking cimetidine.

There may also be hormonal effects. Cimetidine has a weak anti-androgenic action, which means that it can influence the effects of hormones on your body. This can result in impotency and lowered libido or sex drive, and gynaecomastia (enlargement of the breasts in men). This seems to happen more in patients with Zollinger-Ellison syndrome than those who have a simple peptic ulcer.

A number of other side-effects have been reported with cimetidine. Confusion can occur in elderly patients, and skin rashes have also been reported with long-term use. The rash is not very severe and does not last very long, even if treatment is continued. Rarely, other side-effects such as dizziness, diarrhoea or muscle pain have been reported. Again these are not serious but should be reported to your doctor.

Pharmaceutical companies carry out safety tests on all their products, and there is no evidence that cimetidine or any other H_2 antagonist will cause any harm if you are pregnant or breastfeeding. However, because all of these drugs cross the placenta and can usually be excreted in breastmilk, you will probably be advised to avoid taking cimetidine if you are pregnant or breastfeeding unless absolutely necessary.

RANITIDINE

Ranitidine, better known as Zantac, was the second H_2 antagonist to become commercially available to people with peptic ulcer disease. Zantac is available in tablets, granules and syrup form. A single dose can suppress acid secretion for up to 12 hours. The usual dose is around 150 mg twice a day, morning and evening. Some people find they can take the entire dose of 300 mg at night and it is equally effective. You may find this method of dosing more convenient, and this may help to ensure that you finish the course of treatment.

The course of treatment is usually four weeks. You may then go back to your doctor to discuss your condition. Often you will be given an additional four weeks of treatment to ensure that the ulcer is healed. As with cimetidine, prolonging the treatment in this way increases the healing rate of duodenal ulcers.

How Effective Is It?

Ranitidine has a highly significant ulcer-healing rate. Studies have shown that it provides about 80 per cent healing rate for patients with duodenal ulcers, compared with 31 per cent in people taking a placebo (or dummy pill). Recurrence of the ulcer is prevented by long-term treatment with a half-dose (150 mg), to be taken at bedtime.

A number of trials have been performed looking at both cimetidine and ranitidine. The figures are fairly close. One large study of over 1,200 patients found the healing rate for duodenal ulcers was 76 per cent for ranitidine and 70 per cent for cimetidine. One added benefit of ranitidine is that it also increases the healing rate of gastric ulcers, although there is less evidence regarding gastric ulcers.

Side-effects

Ranitidine is remarkably well tolerated by most patients, and rarely causes any major side-effects. Unlike cimetidine, it does not interact with other drugs. It is probably the best treatment for patients who need to take medication such as anticonvulsants or anticoagulants at the same time as their ulcer treatment.

Ranitidine has less of an anti-androgenic activity, so it is less likely to lead to any hormone-related effects such as impotence, lowered sex drive, or gynaecomastia, although occasionally this last side-effect has been reported.

However, there have been some minor side-effects noted. These include skin rash, headache, dizziness and, in the elderly (though rarely), confusion and hallucination. These side-effects tend to affect less than 5 per cent of patients. However, almost the same number of patients reported these symptoms when given a placebo.

As with most drugs, the safety of using ranitidine in pregnancy and breastfeeding has not yet been completely established. For this reason you should avoid taking the drug during these times unless you have discussed it thoroughly with your doctor.

FAMOTIDINE

Famotidine is the newest of the H_2 antagonists; its prescription name is Pepcid. It comes in tablet form, in two doses of either 20 mg or 40 mg.

As with most other H$_2$ antagonists, you do not need to take famotidine on an empty stomach, as the absorption of the drug is not affected by having food in your stomach.

For patients with duodenal or stomach ulcers, the recommended dose is one 40-mg tablet at night before you go to bed. Treatment should continue for about four to eight weeks; for most patients healing is achieved within four weeks. If healing has not occurred by this time, a further four-week period of treatment can be given.

To prevent the recurrence of duodenal ulcers, a reduced dose of 20 mg of famotidine (that is, one tablet a night), is recommended.

How Effective Is It?
Pepcid's action lasts a long time. Clinical trials have shown that a single 40-mg dose reduces gastric acid secretion for at least 10 hours. However, because it has not been on the market for as long as either cimetidine or ranitidine, there have not been as many large-scale trials.

Side-effects
In controlled studies famotidine has been shown to be fairly well tolerated and causes few side-effects. Rarely, headache, dizziness, constipation and diarrhoea have been reported. Even less frequently, side-effects such as dry mouth, nausea and/or vomiting, abdominal discomfort or fatigue have been noted.

As yet no important drug interactions have been identified. So far, drugs which have been tested in humans include warfarin, theophylline, phenytoin and diazepam, among others. It is worth noting that, as mentioned above, some other H$_2$ antagonists such as cimetidine do interact with a number of these drugs.

Famotidine is not recommended for use in pregnancy and should only be prescribed for pregnant women if clearly needed. Because famotidine can be secreted in human milk, breast-feeding mothers who wish to continue with treatment should stop breastfeeding, or alternatively they can stop taking the drug while they are nursing and continue again with treatment when they have weaned their baby.

NIZATIDINE

Nizatidine, or Axid, was launched in 1987. It is very similar to the other H_2 antagonists, and works in much the same way. Nizatidine comes in capsule form in two doses, either 150 mg or 300 mg. The usual recommended dose is 300 mg in the evening. Some people prefer to take a divided dose – 150 mg in the morning and another 150 mg in the evening. A course of treatment usually lasts one month.

To help keep ulcers healed and to prevent a recurrence, the recommended maintenance dose is 150 mg in the evening; treatment may continue for a year.

How Effective Is It?

In clinical trials, nizatidine, as the other H_2 antagonists, significantly reduced acid production and secretion. It also eased ulcer-related symptoms such as pain within the first week of therapy. In most cases up to 80 per cent of ulcers will heal after four weeks of treatment, and up to 90 per cent after a longer course of eight weeks of treatment.

Side-effects

The healing effects of nizatidine are not affected by eating food or taking medications such as antacids. So you can take it at any time and it will work equally well.

Nizatidine has not been on the market as long as drugs such as cimetidine. So far there is no evidence that it interacts with other medications such as warfarin, diazepam and phenytoin, as do some of the other H_2 antagonists.

Because nizatidine is partially metabolized by the liver and excreted by the kidneys, it may not be the best choice for people with impaired kidney or liver function.

In some large-scale trials on nizatidine it was found that side-effects such as anaemia, sweating and urticaria (hives) were more common in people taking the drug than in those who were given placebos (dummy pills). There have also been rare reports of dermatitis, fever, nausea, rashes and mental confusion (this last was reported primarily in elderly patients).

In trials, nizatidine did not appear to have any significant anti-androgenic effects, as does cimetidine. This means it is much less likely to cause hormonal side-effects such as impotence or loss of libido. There have been occasional reports of gynaecomastia (breast enlargement in men) which could have been connected with the use of nizatidine.

And as with the other H_2 antagonists, it is best to avoid taking nizatidine during pregnancy and while breastfeeding.

Case Study – H_2 Antagonists

I've had a duodenal ulcer off and on for around ten years now. A friend mentioned to me about Helicobacter pylori, and I wanted to find out if this could be causing my ulcer.

I asked my doctor to refer me for an endoscopy, which he was happy to do. I was pleased because I thought that if this was the cause, I could be cured once and for all. When they performed the endoscopy I couldn't believe it. They did a biopsy and found that I'm one of the few people with a duodenal ulcer who isn't infected with HP. So we have no idea what caused it. And at the same time they also found I have a second ulcer, quite near the first one.

I'm real lucky because Tagamet works like a dream for me. It completely shuts down the pain. When I've got a flare-up, I take it twice a day, in the morning and evening. The pain usually eases up within a week, but typically it takes about a month to heal my ulcer completely. Unfortunately it always seems to come back within about six to ten months. And I often find that if I'm under a lot of pressure at work it seems to bring it back quicker, but this could be just my imagination.

I'd love to be able to go for longer periods between flare-ups. I'm thinking about asking my doctor if it's safe to take Tagamet for more than four weeks at a go, which is what I usually do. That way it might keep the ulcers healed for a longer period, and they won't give me so much trouble.

EDDIE, 40

WHEN ULCERS DON'T HEAL

Some ulcers do not heal after a course of treatment with H_2 antagonists. In trials this figure ranges from about 10 to 25 per cent. The reasons for this are not clear.

It's possible that compliance, or your willingness to take a medication as instructed, plays a small part. It's also possible that some ulcers heal at a slower rate than others, and that longer courses of treatment may be required, especially if a patient is taking NSAIDs (for arthritis, for example) at the same time.

Another suggestion is that some people's systems may absorb less of a medication than others' do, so that the healing effects are diluted. However, some studies have disproved this theory. Another possibility is that some people's parietal (acid-producing) cells have a reduced sensitivity to some of the H_2 antagonists. How this would work and whether it is actually a fact are still unclear.

Proton Pump Inhibitors

Along with H$_2$ antagonists, an entirely new type of drug has been developed to treat peptic ulcers. Called proton pump inhibitors because they work by stopping the pump that pushes hydrochloric acid out of the parietal cell, they are designed specifically to help prevent the stomach from secreting acid. Research was initially begun on this type of drug because inhibiting gastric acid secretion was known to help heal ulcers and reduce acid-related symptoms.

In the 1970s it was recognized that the cause of ulcers was associated with the stomach producing too much acid. This led to the development of the H$_2$ antagonists, which work by switching off acid secretion. However, even when treatment is successful, a significant number of healed ulcers recur within a year. So pharmaceutical companies began trying to develop drugs that would provide a more powerful inhibiting action, and so proton pump inhibitors were born.

OMEPRAZOLE

The first proton pump inhibitor to be licensed in the UK was omeprazole, which is marketed under the trade name of Losec. Currently it is the most powerful drug of its kind. Omeprazole was first approved in 1989 for the short-term treatment of peptic ulcers which had proved unresponsive to H$_2$ antagonist therapy.

If your doctor does prescribe Losec, chances are you will be taking the recommended dose of one 20-mg capsule a day. For most patients this provides reliable acid control. If this does not work, the dose can safely be increased to 40 mg once a day to achieve greater acid control. You can take the capsules either in the morning or the evening. Another bonus of omeprazole is that the drug is not affected by what you eat or if you take antacids. This means it is still effectively absorbed even if you take it on a full stomach.

HOW EFFECTIVE IS IT?

In appropriate doses, omeprazole can stop the stomach from making any acid for up to 24 hours. Studies have shown that, over a 24-hour period, Losec can dramatically reduce acid production (by 80 to 90 per cent).

Since it is much stronger than other remedies, it can usually heal gastric and duodenal ulcers more quickly. It is estimated that Losec heals about 95 per cent of duodenal ulcers within about four weeks of treatment, compared to about 80 per cent when using H_2 antagonists. And pain is relieved quickly, too – usually after two or three days of treatment. With H_2 antagonists most people (about 80 per cent) find it takes about a week for their pain to disappear.

SIDE-EFFECTS

Omeprazole rarely produces any side-effects. However, it can occasionally affect the metabolism of other drugs you may be taking. Omeprazole can interact with the tranquillizer diazepam and also with the drugs warfarin and phenytoin. So your doctor will need to decide whether omeprazole is the correct medication for you if you are taking these other drugs.

It has been noted that skin rashes, photosensitivity, urticaria and pruritis (itchy skin) can occasionally occur. Diarrhoea and headache can sometimes be severe enough that you will need to stop treatment. And other digestive disturbances have been reported, including constipation, nausea, vomiting and wind. Because it eliminates most gastric acidity, patients taking omeprazole may be more prone to bouts of food poisoning.

Although there are no known dangers of taking omeprazole when pregnant or breastfeeding, this should always be discussed with your doctor. The drug can cross the placenta and also get into the baby's system through the breastmilk.

LANSOPRAZOLE

Another proton pump inhibitor has been marketed under the name Zoton. It works in much the same way as omeprazole, and is similarly effective.

Zoton comes in capsules containing 30 mg of lansoprazole. Taking a single dose inhibits the parietal cells from producing acid by about 80 per cent.

The recommended dose for duodenal ulcers is 30 mg lansoprazole once a day for four weeks. For treatment of gastric ulcers, this dose should be continued daily for eight weeks. For best results it is recommended that lansoprazole is taken in the morning before breakfast.

Other Drugs

In addition to antacids, H_2 antagonists and proton pump inhibitors, there are a number of anti-ulcer drugs available. They work in different ways, and have different functions, than the drugs already mentioned.

Mucosal protective medications are one example. These work to protect the stomach's mucous lining from the effects of acid. Unlike H_2 antagonists and proton pump inhibitors, these protective agents do not inhibit the release of stomach acid. Instead they shield the stomach's mucous lining from being damaged by the acid. The two most commonly prescribed are sucralfate and misoprostol.

SUCRALFATE

This drug is a compound of sucrose aluminium sulphate. It was initially developed as a pepsin inhibitor, to prevent the release of pepsin into the stomach and thereby prevent its effects on the ulcer.

Sucralfate has other potential ulcer-healing benefits. It increases the blood flow to the mucosal lining of the stomach, which aids healing. It increases the secretion of bicarbonate in the stomach, which works as the body's natural antacid, neutralizing stomach acids. It also stimulates the manufacture of prostaglandins, and encourages the growth of healthy new cells.

The usual dose of sucralfate is 1 gram four times a day (an hour before each meal and another dose at night). In clinical trials sucralfate has generally healed duodenal ulcers at around the same rate as H_2 antagonists.

The only common side-effect with this drug is constipation; a fibre-rich diet or laxatives can easily prevent this from becoming a problem.

MISOPROSTOL

Prostaglandins are naturally-occurring chemicals that help to inhibit the secretion of gastric acid. It is thought they have protective effects in ulcer treatment by either inhibiting acid secretion or shielding and protecting the mucosal lining of the stomach.

A drug called misoprostol works in the same way as natural prostaglandins. It stimulates the secretion of bicarbonate and mucus in the stomach. The bicarb helps to neutralize the effects of stomach acid and the mucus helps provide a protective coating over the ulcerated area. This gives it a chance to heal. It also increases blood flow to the tissues in the area. Again, this helps the ulcerated area to heal.

To heal ulcers, about 800 mg of misoprostol is taken each day, usually in divided doses rather than all at once. Studies have shown that it heals ulcers about as effectively as H_2 antagonists after four weeks of treatment. However, it was also found that it did not provide pain relief for duodenal ulcers as effectively as H$_2$ antagonists.

Side-effects

Misoprostol can cause uterine contractions, and for this reason is not to be taken in pregnancy. It can also cause heavier periods and low blood pressure, so if you currently suffer from either of these conditions, you should be sure to mention it to your doctor.

However, the most frequent side-effect is diarrhoea. The likelihood of this increases the higher your dosage is. Luckily, in most cases you'll need no treatment for this and it settles down on its own.

LIQUORICE DERIVATIVES

Medications derived from liquorice have some ulcer-healing effects. It's not certain exactly why this is true. In some cases it may be due to the stimulation of mucus secretion, which then helps protect the ulcerated area.

Using liquorice is an outdated form of treatment, although it was once fairly widely used. Some alternative or complementary therapists rely on liquorice for the treatment of digestive disturbances.

Eliminating *Helicobacter Pylori*

H. pylori is thought to be responsible for about 95 per cent of all duodenal ulcers, and around 75 to 80 per cent of gastric ulcers. *H. pylori* is a life-long infection if left untreated. Furthermore, you can become reinfected or may be infected with different strains of this bacterium.

There are a number of different drug regimens which can eliminate and eradicate *Helicobacter pylori*. There is so far no one treatment or regime that has been definitely deemed best. Doctors are experimenting with different courses of treatment to find the one that is most effective, causes the least side-effects and is safest for the majority of patients.

GUIDELINES FOR TREATMENT

As yet there are no specific guidelines on the ideal treatment to be used to eliminate *Helicobacter pylori*. There are a number of effective combinations; the one you receive will probably be determined by your general practitioner or specialist.

Most are known as dual or triple therapy, and involve the use of one or two antibiotics along with an anti-ulcer medication (*see pages 87–88*). Studies have shown that mono-therapy – simply giving one antibiotic on its own without an anti-ulcer medication – is not effective.

Some doctors prefer dual therapy, as this cuts down on the number of tablets you need to take, while others prefer triple therapy because some studies have shown this to be most effective. A number of studies and large-scale trials are currently underway to try to identify the ideal combination. Until that time, you will have to rely upon your doctor's advice.

However, a management guide was compiled in March 1995 by a group of nine clinicians representing academic centres, hospitals and general practices from around Britain. It has been circulated to doctors around the UK, and it is hoped that this will offer doctors a framework to consult and work from when treating patients with duodenal ulcers.

The group recommended that for new patients who go to their doctors complaining of symptoms relating to a possible duodenal ulcer, a complete medical history and preliminary investigations should be undertaken. Once it is determined that the patient may be suitable for eradication treatment, he or she should be given a course of either dual or triple therapy.

HOW IT IS DONE

Generally most regimes will require about 14 days of treatment with antibiotics and an anti-secretory drug, or one that reduces the amount of acid your stomach produces (an H_2 antagonist or proton pump inhibitor). As yet, no single eradication method is regarded as being the definitive one. There are various combinations in use, although not all of the components are as yet licensed for use in the treatment of *H. pylori* infection. However, your doctor can use his or her own discretion in deciding which medication to prescribe.

Dual and triple therapy usually requires fairly large numbers of tablets to be taken throughout the day – sometimes as many as 14 or 15. Depending on the drug combinations, you may find that you feel a little queasy or nauseous at times, or suffer from diarrhoea or constipation. You may also notice that your stools have become much darker. These side-effects quickly pass, and you should not just stop taking the tablets. If you find the side-effects difficult to cope with, go back to your doctor. It may be one specific medication that is causing the problem; your doctor can switch you to another similar drug.

However, most of the patients who have been on dual or triple therapy are amazed at how quickly their pain and discomfort clear up, often within about a week or so. The relief is so immediate it is worth persevering even if you do experience some disconcerting side-effects.

Case Study – HP Triple Therapy

My ulcer caused me so much pain, I was in agony. Nothing seemed to help. I took tablets from the doctor and they worked for a while, but the pain would always come back. My GP eventually decided to try eradication therapy. He explained that I might be infected with a bug that causes ulcers. And if this worked, the ulcer should go away and never come back.

I was counting the days until I could start it. I couldn't imagine what it would be like to be free of the pain. I took three different tablets four times a day for two weeks. I took two antibiotics and a third tablet, omeprazole. One of the tablets made me feel a little sick, but I persevered.

Honestly, by the end of the first week of treatment most of the pain had gone. And by the end of the second week, I was totally clear of pain. I couldn't believe it. Although you think of two weeks of suffering, having to take all those tablets. And you can't have any alcohol when you're on the treatment. But it's well worth it.

My ulcer has gone completely now. I haven't had any more trouble, and consider it a great success. When I think of what it has done for me, I'd advise anyone with an ulcer to go for it.

BARBARA, 45

Triple Therapy

The triple therapy combination will typically include three of the following:

- an acid suppressant, such as an H_2 antagonist or a proton pump inhibitor
- a bismuth salt, which helps protect the stomach lining by coating it and also seems to have an anti-*Helicobacter pylori* effect
- a nitromidazole antibiotic, such as metronidazole or tinidazole
- another antibiotic, for example amoxycillin or tetracycline.

Dual Therapy

A dual therapy combination will usually include:

- an acid suppressant, such as an H_2 antagonist or a proton pump inhibitor
- one antibiotic.

TESTING FOR ERADICATION

Once you've been through dual or triple therapy, you will usually need to go back to your doctor or specialist about a month to six weeks after starting treatment. Your doctor will want to find out whether your symptoms have disappeared. He or she may also refer you for testing to see if the *Helicobacter pylori* has been eradicated. This usually involves a simple blood test.

Again, there are no strict guidelines as to whether first-time patients given a course of eradication therapy need to be tested for active infection with *H. pylori* at the end of treatment.

Some doctors will choose the 'wait and see' approach. This means they will not test you, but will wait to see if you develop the symptoms again, which could indicate that the treatment was not a success.

According to respondents to the initial survey put out by the group of nine clinicians mentioned above, GPs generally felt it was more practical to wait and monitor their patients for the reappearance of symptoms.

Other practitioners believe that patients should be tested to see if eradication therapy has indeed been successful. This is particularly relevant among patients who would be put at increased risk if the acid-suppressant therapy was withdrawn.

The most effective way of testing to see if eradication therapy has been a success is to have a repeat endoscopy and biopsy, so the doctor can check to make sure that *H. pylori* is no longer present.

Blood tests work by checking the level of *H. pylori* antibodies in your blood. These antibodies will have been produced by your body to help fight the *H. pylori* infection. However, they can remain in your system for quite some time even after the bacterium itself is no longer present. So antibody tests are not as reliable as biopsies to check whether or not you have a current infection. They are better for the initial diagnosis of whether or not you have ever been infected at some time in the past.

HOW SUCCESSFUL IS ERADICATION?

There have been a number of studies looking at the comparative success rates of dual and triple therapy. Overall, it appears that using either dual or triple therapy seems to eliminate duodenal ulcers in up to 90 per cent of cases. The recurrence rate seems to be approximately 5 to 7 per cent after about one year following treatment.

A number of different factors can affect the success rate of *H. pylori* treatment. Again, the most obvious is patient compliance. Because of the sheer numbers of tablets that you must take with either dual or triple therapy, many patients give up halfway through or do not finish the whole course. Another reason a patient may give up is as a result of the possible minor side-effects.

One study evaluating triple therapy compliance found that taking less than 75 per cent of the course of tablets dramatically reduced the eradication success rate to between only 20 and 50 per cent. So it is crucial that if your doctor gives you a course of medication, you complete the course.

It has also been found that some patients are resistant to treatment with the antibiotic metronidazole, so other antibiotics must be used in its place. It's also suspected that there may be especially strong strains of *H. pylori*, and that some of these are fairly resistant to treatment. It may occasionally take more than one course, trying different antibiotics, until the treatment is completely successful.

WHY ERADICATE?

Taking all these tablets may seem like a lot of effort. So why should doctors consider eradication therapy? The answer is that study after study has shown that if you get rid of the *Helicobacter pylori* infection, the ulcer heals and the majority of people are cured for life. Only about 5 to 7 per cent will develop another ulcer. With H_2 antagonist treatment, it's estimated that around 80 to 90 per cent of ulcers will recur within a year after successful treatment.

IF ERADICATION THERAPY FAILS

If you have been on a course of eradication therapy and it hasn't worked, your doctor has a couple of possible options. One is to prescribe you a second course of treatment. It is likely that your doctor will choose a different combination of drugs, to see if this is more successful. In many cases the second course does the trick.

It's also possible that you may be referred to a hospital gastroenterology department for endoscopy (assuming you have not yet had one). This would confirm the presence of a peptic ulcer and also, if a biopsy is performed, whether you are infected with *Helicobacter pylori*.

After the results of these investigations are in, you and your doctor can then make some decisions about the next stage of your treatment. If could be that you are put on long-term therapy with H_2 antagonists or some other acid-suppressant drug, or, in rare cases, your doctor may discuss with you the possibility of surgery. (*See Chapter 8.*)

Dealing with Relapses

It's likely that you will know someone who has been taking ulcer drugs for many months, or even years, because his or her ulcer seems to keep coming back no matter what treatment or therapy is tried, so he or she has to keep taking the medication. This has always been one of the problems associated with ulcers. Even though they are healed initially, they have a nasty habit of reappearing, often fairly soon after treatment. Most relapses are accompanied by pain and, occasionally, by bleeding or perforation which puts your health at considerable risk.

Some people are more prone to relapses in the first year or two after treatment; this is especially so of heavy smokers. It may be that the effects of cigarette smoking on your ulcer are so strong they cancel out the benefits of the ulcer medication.

There are two ways of treating relapses. Most commonly, each relapse will be treated with an H_2 antagonist for four to eight weeks, a treatment similar to your initial therapy.

Unfortunately, this therapy does not prevent further relapses. So an alternative approach is to keep the ulcers healed by putting you on continuous long-term drug treatment. In most cases this will involve a smaller dose of an H_2 antagonist, usually only needed to be taken once a night. Acid levels in the stomach seem to be greatest in the early morning, when the stomach is empty, so taking the medication at night provides the most protection at the most vulnerable part of the 24-hour period. And all the H_2 antagonists are extremely successful at inhibiting nighttime secretion of acid.

Continuing with long-term therapy has a number of benefits. It helps to keep acid secretion under control, and your
ulcer healed. It can help keep you free of symptoms and reduce
the risk of the potential complications of duodenal ulcers.

You must stick with this treatment. It is known that if treatment is stopped at any time, even for just a few days, there's a
strong possibility your ulcer will recur. Studies have found
that, at present, eight out of ten patients will have a relapse if
long-term treatment is stopped.

There is less information available on the effectiveness of
maintenance therapy for stomach ulcers than for duodenal
ulcers. Most doctors still recommend a maintenance dose for
some patients, while others may adopt a wait and see
approach, to determine if your ulcer is well and truly healed
or if it will return if the treatment is stopped.

Fortunately, with the development of treatment to eradicate *H. pylori* it is hoped that eventually fewer and fewer
patients will be on long-term drug therapy.

What About Surgery?

In the past the standard treatment for peptic ulcers was
antacids. If this didn't work, which it often didn't, the next
step was fairly radical surgical procedures.

Over the past 20 years or so, the number of people having
surgery for uncomplicated ulcers – that is, ulcers with no serious complications such as bleeding – has been declining. This
drop began even before the advent of drugs such as H_2 antagonists; now that they have been developed, surgery is no longer
used in the treatment of uncomplicated ulcer disease. One
study found that in the year following the introduction of H_2
antagonists, the number of elective operations fell by almost
30 per cent. Throughout the 1980s, the number of operations

performed for ulcers around the world fell dramatically (by about 90 per cent).

These days surgery is really only used in medical emergencies such as bleeding or perforations, or in those very rare cases where patients, for some reason, cannot continue with – or refuse to continue with – long-term drug treatment. Even then, most of these patients will need to be young, fit and healthy before elective surgery will be considered. This is because surgery, though effective, can result in irreversible complications (*see Chapter 8*).

8

THE DANGERS OF ULCERS

Peptic ulcers are a serious business. Although many patients themselves take their symptoms lightly, doctors do not. The clinicians are only too aware of the fact that untreated ulcers can lead to serious complications that require emergency surgery. It's thought that around one in 500 patients with peptic ulcer disease will eventually require surgery, usually for either bleeding or perforation, the two most common complications.

Peptic ulcer disease is still of the UK's top killers. There are around 60,000 hospital admissions for complications of ulcers every year. Of these, about 4,500 patients die – more than the number of deaths resulting from either cervical cancer or asthma. The majority of these patients are usually elderly.

Luckily, with treatments improving all the time and better diagnostic techniques and newer surgical methods, the dangerous complications of ulcers can be effectively treated. Treatment often helps prevent a recurrence of the problem and, in many cases, also eliminates the ulcer completely.

In the past, surgery was often performed to treat uncomplicated ulcers, to avoid persistent recurrences or so the patient would not have to undergo long-term medical therapy.

Nowadays, surgery is really only performed to treat the complications of ulcers. And although its role in uncomplicated ulcer disease has diminished dramatically, surgery still has a major part to play in the treatment of bleeding and perforation.

Traditionally, surgery for an ulcer was a major operation. The patient would have to spend quite a time in hospital, and weeks and months recuperating. These types of procedures resulted in uncomfortable and inconvenient side-effects, ranging from minor diarrhoea to the inability to eat more than a little food at a time. And these side-effects were permanent.

In the last five years, however, the development of minimal access surgery or 'keyhole' surgery has meant that similar procedures can be carried out with less scarring and a much quicker recovery time. And, as better and more effective medications for peptic ulcer disease have been developed, the number of people who need emergency surgery is now fairly small. The discovery of the role of *Helicobacter pylori* and effective eradication therapies mean this number is decreasing all the time.

Complications of Ulcers

BLEEDING

This is the most common complication of an ulcer. The walls of the stomach and the duodenum are richly supplied with blood vessels, including both arteries and veins.

If an untreated ulcer slowly erodes into a blood vessel in the lining of the stomach and duodenum, the result is internal bleeding – called a haemorrhage. The vessels begin to bleed into the stomach and digestive tract. This bleeding can be very slow and not easily detectable, especially if only a tiny artery or vein is affected. The first sign may be fatigue and tiredness due to anaemia, which develops because you are slowly losing iron-rich blood.

However, the bleeding may also occur very rapidly, particularly if a larger blood vessel is affected. You may notice dizziness and faintness; this is caused by the reduced blood circulation to the brain. A feeling of fullness in the abdomen is also common, and this is usually following by the vomiting of blood through the mouth – haematemesis – or the passage of copious amounts of blood in the stools, called melaena, or both.

If you vomit blood because of an ulcer, the material often looks like coffee grounds. It consists of a dark, brownish material rather than bright red liquid. This is because the pigment that gives blood its red colour is changed by the stomach acids into a brown pigment.

When blood moves slowly through the digestive tract into the stools, it changes from red to a black, sticky mess, often referred to as 'tarry' stool. It is not just dark, but actually black. Occasionally, due to a swift passage of the blood through the digestive tract, the stools do appear red, but this is less common.

Vomiting blood or passing blood in the stools can be extremely frightening. But it's important to remember that the actual amount of blood lost may be considerably less than it appears.

It's also important to remember that black stools can be caused by taking certain medications (including iron tablets) and even some foods and drinks, such as Guinness. Your doctor may perform a test on the stool, called a faecal occult blood test. This test can detect the presence of iron in the stool, which is an indication of bleeding. But there can be many reasons for iron in the stool; your doctor will then need to determine the cause, for instance if you have been taking aspirin, eating certain foods or taking other medications. He or she will probably ask you a number of questions about your diet and lifestyle to try to determine the reason you have a positive test result.

Never underestimate the dangers of a bleeding ulcer, especially if you haemorrhage quite suddenly. It's estimated that if you have a bleeding ulcer, your risk of dying is between 4 and 10 per cent if it is not treated immediately.

So, if you have a history of peptic ulcer disease and you notice any of these symptoms, it is absolutely vital that you seek medical attention right away. Most people with bleeding ulcers require hospital treatment. You should either call your doctor or get yourself to the casualty department of your local hospital.

The doctors may ask you questions about your medical history as well as what other medications you may be taking. Certain drugs, such as aspirin and NSAIDs, can cause minor bleeding and affect the body's blood-clotting mechanisms. Usually an endoscopy will be performed as soon as possible after your arrival in hospital. This is done to determine the site of the bleeding and also whether it has stopped on its own or not.

In about nine out of ten cases of bleeding ulcers, the bleeding will stop on its own without treatment. It can persist or recur, however. If this is the case, you may need emergency surgery. Depending on a number of different factors, for example your overall condition, how severe the bleeding is, how severe your ulcer is, and whether you have had episodes of bleeding in the past, the doctors will then determine which operation is best for you.

Case Study – Bleeding

About two years ago I started having dizzy spells and feeling breathless. It got progressively worse, until finally I had to call out the doctor one day. He came to the house and asked me a lot about my symptoms, and examined me, but couldn't find anything wrong. At the time he didn't ask me about my stools. I didn't mention to him that they were virtually black, because I thought it was something to do with what I'd been eating.

The next day I went to have a blood test, and when the results came back they said I was severely anaemic and would have to go into hospital as soon as possible. When I got to hospital I was feeling worse and worse. I could barely get up the stairs, and was on the verge of completely passing out. They put me in a wheelchair because I couldn't walk upright, and finally I lay on the bed, afraid to sit up because I felt so bad.

I needed a blood and platelet transfusion, and we waited around four hours for it to arrive by taxi. After the transfusion I started feeling better fairly quickly. I stayed in hospital, and the next day had an endoscopy. I had a general anaesthetic for this, and found out later it was because they suspected I had a bleeding ulcer and wanted to seal off the bleeding vessels.

When I saw my doctor again he told me how serious my condition had been. He gave me some tablets for the ulcer, which made me feel dizzy and unwell. He's changed my medication, and it now seems to be working. I don't take them all the time — only when the symptoms come on. One of the problems is that whenever I feel unwell I relate it to my ulcer. Just recently I was feeling tired and sick, with a constant feeling of dizziness and nausea. I naturally thought it was my ulcer playing up. In fact, when I went to see the doctor I found I had measles!

RICHARD, 31

Symptoms and Signs

- abdominal fullness and discomfort
- dizziness and feeling lightheaded
- fatigue and lethargy
- vomiting of brown material that looks like coffee grounds
- passage of black, tarry-looking stools.

PERFORATION

This condition is less common than bleeding. It is equally if not more serious, however. A perforated ulcer requires immediate medical attention and surgery, and must be treated as a medical emergency. It can be fatal within about 48 hours if emergency treatment is not given. Many of the deaths from ulcers occur as a result of perforation.

A perforation occurs when the ulcer erodes a hole right through the wall of the stomach or duodenum. This, in turn, can lead to peritonitis, an inflammation and infection of the peritoneum, the membrane that lines the abdominal cavity. Peritonitis occurs because the acid and food leaking through a perforated stomach ulcer, or the bile from a duodenal ulcer, can irritate and inflame the peritoneum. Chemical inflammation of this kind is usually soon followed by bacterial infection.

A perforated ulcer usually causes very severe, very sudden abdominal pain. This is because the abdominal muscles over and around the area will tighten, as muscles over an inflamed area normally do. You may find your whole abdomen is extremely painful. If a large area of the peritoneum is inflamed, you can even go into shock. Your blood pressure will suddenly drop because of the lowered volume of blood circulating around the body. Symptoms of shock usually include sweating, pallor and pale skin, cold and clammy skin and a rapid pulse.

Fortunately, the pain and symptoms of perforation are usually so severe that most patients do call their doctor or hospital almost immediately. This allows for emergency surgery to be carried out as quickly as possible.

Once you are at the casualty department, the diagnosis of a perforated ulcer can be confirmed using a simple abdominal X-ray. If the diagnosis is confirmed, surgery can be performed without delay.

Symptoms and Signs

- severe abdominal pain
- shock
- pallor
- cold, clammy skin
- rapid pulse.

OBSTRUCTION

If an ulcer occurs in or around the pylorus (the narrow outlet at the lower end of the stomach), the pylorus can become swollen and scarred. This in turn can lead to a blockage in the pyloric canal – a condition known as pyloric stenosis. With the development of effective treatments for peptic ulcers, obstruction rarely occurs nowadays.

Pyloric stenosis prevents both the gastric juices and partially-digested food and liquid from passing into the duodenum. Instead, all this material accumulates and builds up in the stomach. Sometimes the stomach is able to stretch and distend enough to hold a few litres of fluid, but eventually it will be so full that you need to vomit the undigested food. Before this happens you may notice a feeling of fullness and bloat, and also nausea. You may also feel pain and discomfort.

Repeated vomiting is usually the main symptom of pyloric stenosis. If it is left untreated, the loss of body fluids and the lack of food absorption can lead to you becoming dehydrated and malnourished.

This kind of blockage doesn't occur overnight. It usually affects people who have a history of ulcers (over at least five years) rather than those who have just developed an ulcer.

The diagnosis of pyloric stenosis can easily be confirmed by a barium meal X-ray or endoscopy. Treatment usually involves emptying the stomach using a tube that is inserted through your nose and down your throat into your stomach. This emptying process may take several days. During this time you'll be given fluid and nutrients directly into your bloodstream through an intravenous drip.

Depending on the severity of the obstruction, surgery may also be needed. This usually involves opening the abdominal cavity (while the patient is under general anaesthesia) and making an incision into the pylorus to create an extra-wide passage for food. Sometimes, however, simply healing the ulcer using anti-ulcer medications reduces the swelling sufficiently to reopen the pyloric canal and allow the passage of food.

Symptoms and Signs

- bloating
- nausea
- abdominal pain and discomfort
- repeated vomiting.

Treating Complications

In the past, many ulcer patients voluntarily underwent surgery to treat or cure their ulcers. These days routine surgery is no longer performed, and in fact has virtually disappeared as a method of treatment in the UK. However, surgery is still performed to treat the emergency complications of peptic ulcers.

GASTRECTOMY

This is the oldest, and now least widely performed operation for treating ulcer complications. A gastrectomy involves removing a portion of the stomach where the ulcer is located, which is usually the same area in which the bleeding or perforation has occurred.

Partial gastrectomy was the operation most commonly performed. This involved removing the lower part of the stomach – the antrum – where most of the acid-stimulating hormone gastrin is produced. So in effect this operation helped to decrease excess acid production, often a cause of ulcers, as well as removing the ulcer itself.

One reason this operation has fallen out of favour is that it led to debilitating side-effects. Gastrectomy often made patients virtually life-long cripples. They usually suffered diarrhoea, had to go for the 'little and often' approach to food, and needed to avoid drinking any fluid with their meals. The development of effective drugs that inhibit acid secretion has, fortunately, made this type of surgery almost a thing of the past.

VAGOTOMY

Vagotomy involves cutting or severing the vagus nerve, which runs from the brain down to the stomach. This nerve is responsible for the stimulation of acid secretion and production. By cutting this nerve, the amount of gastric acid produced is reduced by about 60 per cent.

There are different types of vagotomy, although most of the variations have never gained wide acceptance or popularity. In a truncal vagotomy, the branches are cut just where they enter the abdomen through the diaphragm. This affects the nerve fibres that supply not only the stomach, but the other abdominal organs as well. In selective vagotomy, only those nerve fibres supplying the stomach are cut.

All types of vagotomy decrease the output of stomach acid. However, there are significant complications associated with this operation. Because the vagus nerve allows the stomach to empty into the duodenum after a meal, cutting it alters the

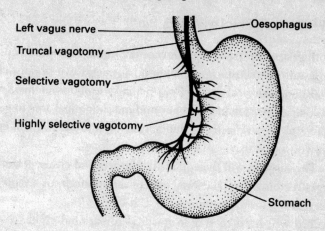

Left vagus nerve

Truncal vagotomy

Selective vagotomy

Highly selective vagotomy

Oesophagus

Stomach

The Vagus Nerve and Where It Is Cut

normal functioning of the stomach. As a result, side-effects include diarrhoea and the inability to eat more than a very small meal at any one sitting. To prevent this, the surgeons perform a drainage procedure at the same time as the vagotomy. This procedure is called a pyloroplasty, in which the normally narrow pylorus is surgically enlarged. When these operations are combined they are often referred to as 'vagotomy and drainage' or 'vagotomy and pyloroplasty'. Even with the drainage procedure, about 20 per cent of patients will be left with some problems; of these, 5 per cent will suffer quite serious ones.

Both of these older operations, gastrectomy and vagotomy (and their variations) are still occasionally performed to treat the complications of ulcers. Because these complications are medical emergencies, the operation you have will depend very much on your local hospital and the surgical ability of the doctors on staff at the time.

What Surgery Involves

Both gastrectomy and vagotomy operations will require you to be admitted to hospital and undergo a general anaesthetic. The traditional surgical method of opening the abdomen involves making an incision in the upper midline abdominal area to gain access to the stomach and duodenum. As a result you will end up with a scar that is about 18 cm (6 in) long.

The surgeon will then go inside the area and either perform a gastrectomy, and take away part of the stomach, or a vagotomy, cutting the vagus nerve.

You will need to stay in hospital for around eight to ten days. Once you are home you will usually need about six to 12 weeks to recover. You will probably need to avoid moderate lifting for about six weeks, and heavy lifting for three months. This gives your abdominal scar a chance to heal.

Newer Techniques

Nowadays most gastric surgeons prefer to avoid these major operations. Instead they tend simply to stitch up the bleeding vessel or close or plug the hole of the perforation. They do not attempt to 'cure' the ulcer through surgery or take out more of the digestive tract than is absolutely necessary.

Although these procedures are much less radical, your surgeon may still choose to obtain access to your abdominal organs in the traditional way – by an incision in your abdomen. If this is the case, you will still undergo a general anaesthetic, but the stitching (of the bleeding vessel) or closing (of the perforation) are much simpler procedures. To treat bleeding, the surgeon will insert a few stitches to seal off the blood vessel. To treat perforation, the surgeon will pull the hole to close it, then tie a bit of fat over so it seals the perforation.

You will probably spend around five to seven days in hospital, and four to six weeks recuperating at home. There are usually no side-effects or complications after this type of surgery.

KEYHOLE SURGERY

Within the last five years or so keyhole surgical techniques for ulcer surgery have been developed. There are a number of benefits to this type of procedure. If you undergo keyhole surgery you have a much smaller, almost minimal scar because the incision is smaller and the instruments are so tiny. And you will recover more quickly.

An increasing number of patients around Britain are being offered keyhole surgery for treating complications of ulcers. However, it is still uncommon and fairly unusual to have this type of surgery. It is more often offered in specialist centres.

Keyhole, or laparascopic surgery, is only performed to treat a perforated ulcer – it is not used for bleeding ulcers. A laparascope is inserted into the abdomen, and a tiny telescope sent down through the tube. This allows the surgeon to see what is going on in the area.

Through other incisions nearby, the surgeon will insert tiny instruments with which to perform the operation. He or she will then stitch up the hole and plug it with fat to prevent it opening, and to seal it up.

After keyhole surgery to close a perforation you will spend around three to four days in hospital, and around two weeks recuperating. In most cases you can take up your normal activities as soon as you feel fit enough to do so.

ENDOSCOPIC SURGERY

Using endoscopes to perform surgery is an even newer technique than keyhole surgery. It has made surgery for ulcer complications even safer and easier, though not every surgeon is trained in the technique.

Endoscopic surgery is only suitable for treating bleeding ulcers – it is not used for treating perforations. Unlike traditional or keyhole surgery, for which you need a general anaesthetic, you will only be given a local anaesthetic or mild sedative for endoscopic surgery.

The surgeon will insert an endoscope, and will inject the bleeding vessel through the endoscope with saline, water or adrenaline. In some cases the surgeon uses chemicals called sclerosants, which are used for the treatment of varicose veins. Injecting these solutions acts to shut down the bleeding vessel, virtually closing it off.

This procedure is often performed at the same time as an endoscopy to diagnose an ulcer. If the doctor sees signs that the ulcer is bleeding or has recently bled, it is now common and widespread to treat the bleeding at the same time. This helps to prevent you from needing a major operation at a later date. However, if endoscopic sclerotherapy does not work, or if you have one or more bleeds, or re-bleed, you may need to have open surgery.

At a few selected centres around the UK, some surgeons are using lasers inserted down the endoscope to seal off bleeding vessels. Again, this is not at all common, though as more doctors are trained in the technique it may become more widespread.

After endoscopic surgery you will be asked to stay in hospital for around 48 to 72 hours so that the surgeons can monitor your condition and ensure that the bleeding has stopped. Once you are home, you will need around one to two weeks to recuperate and convalesce.

Care after Surgery

Depending on the type of surgery you have had, you may need to take quite some time to recuperate and get your strength back. If you have had abdominal surgery, you will need about six to 12 weeks to recover. Procedures such as keyhole surgery require only about two weeks' recovery time.

Although these procedures will treat any complications, they will not treat or cure your ulcer. So once the life-saving procedures have been performed it is likely that you will be given eradication therapy if it is suspected or shown that you are infected with *Helicobacter pylori*. This consists of either dual or triple therapy to eliminate any infection (*see Chapter* 7).

Once eradication therapy has been successful it is very unlikely that your ulcer will return. The current figures indicate that only around 5 per cent of patients will have a relapse or recurrence after eradication therapy. However, if eradication therapy is not given, even after an operation such as vagotomy there is a recurrence rate of around 15 per cent.

In the past doctors often issued very strong guidelines on taking care of yourself after having surgery for ulcers. For example, you may have been advised to stick to a bland diet, avoiding spicy foods, and to stop drinking alcohol. You may have been advised to get a lot of bed rest, and avoid exerting yourself. Although these guidelines no longer hold true, it's likely that some doctors, and certainly many patients, believe that they must face some restrictions after having ulcer surgery.

There is no need to follow any special diet or eating programme. As with any major operation, at the hospital you should be given some specific guidelines, either verbally or in written form, to follow during your recuperation period. For instance you may need to avoid driving for a period of time after surgery, and obviously to avoid heavy lifting or activities that may put stress and strain on your scar. But in most cases you will be free to eat and drink what you please.

If you are a smoker, there is little doubt that it is highly advisable that you make sincere efforts to stop. Smoking not only plays a part in the development of the initial ulcer, but is also a well-known contributor to complications and recurrences of ulcers. Cigarette smoking also impairs the body's ability to heal itself after injury, which means that you may take much longer to recuperate after any surgical procedure. For advice on ways to give up smoking, see Chapter 9.

9

HELPING YOURSELF

If you're a sufferer of peptic ulcers it is a good idea to start paying attention to your lifestyle and starting to make some healthier changes. This will help improve your all-round health, even if it does not have a direct effect on your ulcer.

One of the problems with persistent conditions such as ulcers is that they can wear you down. Feeling unwell, taking regular medications and having to make repeated visits to the doctor can take their toll. They can sap your energy and make you see yourself as an unhealthy person.

The best way to overcome this feeling of being 'ill' is to take better care of yourself. This will improve not only your physical well-being but also improve you emotionally and mentally. It can help you change your outlook on your condition, and also help you to deal better with any problems that arise as a result of your condition.

Advice from Your Doctor

With all the new evidence about the causes of ulcers, and the ever-improving treatments that are available, doctors rarely offer specific lifestyle advice to patients with ulcers. The days of recommending bed rest and bland diets are thankfully, long gone.

Study after study has shown that many factors you may think affect your ulcer, such as your diet, in fact do not. This does not mean that certain triggers — too much alcohol or fatty foods, for example — will not bring on the pain of an ulcer attack.

Each person must decide for him- or herself what approach works best. You should discuss with your doctor various ideas and suggestions. This way the two of you can work out a program that suits you.

Taking Care of Yourself

DIET

Though there's little evidence that what you eat can cause an ulcer, there's no doubt that once you've developed one, certain foods can make it worse or better.

Many people with ulcers suspect or complain that spicy or hot foods bring on their symptoms. In fact there is no clinical evidence that spicy foods affect ulcers, but if you find that eating curries or spicy foods brings on pain and discomfort, don't eat them. There is also no evidence that coffee or tea makes symptoms worse. But again, if you find that these bother you, give them up.

Milk and milk-containing products are thought to coat the stomach, and can relieve the pain of an ulcer. It is thought that the milk also helps to neutralize the effects of gastric acid, so drinking a glass can ease any pain, especially pain that occurs at night.

You may also find that if you go for long periods between meals your ulcer pain flares up. If this is the case, consider eating 'little and often'.

Some patients find that highly acidic foods like citrus juices cause a problem, while others find that rich or fatty foods aggravate their symptoms. Fats and oils can in fact help slow down acid production; nevertheless many sufferers find that rich, creamy foods give them problems. It will probably be a matter of trial and error to find out which foods give you grief.

There is now evidence that increasing your fibre intake, for instance by eating more whole-grain bread and cereals, fruit and vegetables can help prevent a recurrence of a duodenal ulcer. So if you have (or used to have) a duodenal ulcer, increase your fibre intake.

ALCOHOL

There is some evidence that drinking alcohol can aggravate the pain of an already-existing ulcer. It's thought that the alcohol hitting the raw, open crater that is an ulcer is what causes the pain. This may not, however, apply to every type of alcohol. Some people find spirits make the ulcer painful, while others find that red wine brings it on.

You are the only one who will know what to avoid. When it comes to drinking, you should always stick to the recommended guidelines. That is, no more than two to three units per day for women or three to four units per day for men. A unit is one glass of wine, one measure of spirits, or half a pint of beer or lager.

It's also a good idea to avoid overloading your system by going on a binge. Try to spread your units throughout the week, and try to have a couple of drink-free days each week.

If you have a drink problem and find it difficult to stick to these limits, organizations such as Alcohol Concern can help. You'll find their address in the Useful Addresses section (*see* page 126).

SMOKING

Although smoking is not healthy for anyone, it is even more damaging to people with peptic ulcer disease. Study after study has shown that cigarette smoking impairs the healing of ulcers, which means they will heal at a slower rate. This is true even in patients taking effective anti-ulcer medication such as H_2 antagonists. Smoking cigarettes also increases the risk of your ulcer recurring. A new study has also shown that cigarette smokers are more likely to be infected with *Helicobacter pylori*, the bacterium thought to be responsible for a large majority of ulcers.

Nobody believes that giving up smoking is easy, and you may need help in doing this. There are a number of options open to you. QUIT is an organization that helps people stop smoking. They have a number of leaflets and can also refer to you local stop-smoking services. Their address and phone number are given in the Useful Addresses section (*see page 126*).

Some people find that joining a stop-smoking group provides them with the encouragement they need to give up. Others may find that something like nicotine patches are the answer to helping them with withdrawal symptoms. There are also a number of aids such as herbal cigarettes or dummy cigarettes as well as complementary treatments such as hypnotherapy and acupuncture, which have all been used in various ways to help smokers kick the habit.

However, evidence from QUIT indicates that, in fact, the majority of people give up without any outside help at all, and that having the motivation and desire to quit seems to be the key to becoming a non-smoker. Knowing that it will improve your health and the state of your ulcer disease should help provide some motivation.

REDUCING STRESS LEVELS

While stress has not been shown to be a cause of ulcers, it is suspected that high stress levels can contribute to a number of digestive disturbances, and may make ulcer symptoms worse. Many patients report that they develop symptoms during periods of long-term stress, though clinical trials offer no proof that ulcers recur when life gets particularly stressful.

It is thought that stress may aggravate the pain of an ulcer or create indigestion that is associated with ulcers, but experts have no proof that stress is an important factor in the development of ulcers.

Some doctors have noted that ulcer flare-ups seem to be more frequent during the week, and less so on the weekend and Monday. One interesting study found that there was an increase in reported cases of perforated ulcers during the heavy air raids of the Second World War.

In spite of the conflicting evidence, it's likely that we could all benefit from a reduction in stress. Luckily there are many ways you can do this.

Stress-reduction Techniques

There are any number of ways to reduce your stress levels. Regular exercise, a healthy diet and time for yourself every day can go a long way to easing anxiety and pressure.

The following relaxation technique takes only about five minutes, and can easily be done at home. Studies have shown that a simple method such as this slows your breathing and pulse rate, lowers blood pressure and provides a temporary respite from the hustle and bustle all around you.

Five-step Relaxation Technique

1 Find a quiet place and sit or lie down comfortably.
   Make sure it's somewhere you won't be interrupted.
2 Close your eyes and be aware of your body. Try to avoid
   thinking about problems or chores. Instead, concentrate
   on areas of muscular tension. Relax those parts, such as
   your shoulders and neck.
3 Notice how you are breathing. Breathe through your nose,
   focusing on each breath. Relax your mouth and let your
   tongue fall from away from the roof of your mouth.
4 Allow your breaths to become deeper, longer and slower.
   Make sure you are breathing from your abdomen, not your
   chest. When your mind wanders, which is natural, bring it
   back to concentrate on your breathing.
5 After about five minutes, end this relaxation exercise
   the way you began. Gently begin to stir, open your
   eyes, and sit or stand carefully. You should feel relaxed
   and refreshed.

Initially you may find it difficult to shut off the outside world
and concentrate on yourself. But as you get more experienced, you will find that you can relax in as little as five minutes a day. Initially you can do this technique for as long a time
and as often as you feel you need to. As you begin to feel better you can reduce the number of sessions. You may find that
simply doing this a few times a week is more than enough.

Creative Visualization

This uses your mind and brain to conjure up images that are
pleasant and relaxing. It is easy to learn and can be done almost
anywhere at any time.

- Find a quiet place where you can sit or lie down undisturbed. Close your eyes, and start to breathe slowly and deeply.
- Try to clear your mind of worries or other concerns.
- Imagine you are in a peaceful place, for instance at the seaside or in the mountains.
- Get a clear image of what this peaceful place is like. Imagine how it sounds, looks, feels and smells. Continue with your measured breathing.
- As the picture becomes more real to you, you will find yourself relaxing and you will feel less tense and stressed.
- You can stay in this place for as long as you wish. When you feel relaxed, slowly bring yourself back to the present. Imagine yourself leaving your peaceful place and coming back to where you are located. Slowly open your eyes and stand or sit up gently. You should now feel relaxed and refreshed.

YOGA

Yoga has been practised for over 6,000 years. It is a combination of exercise positions (called 'asanas') and breathing techniques. By combining these two techniques, yoga has been shown to help with relaxation and stress reduction. It is also good for asthma, stress-related conditions, digestive disorders, headache and depression.

Most yoga classes last around 60 to 90 minutes so that you have time to receive their full benefit. Few of us have the time to take a class every day, but many of the positions and breathing techniques can easily be practised at home. There are also a number of yoga videocassettes for sale, which again allow you to practise at home.

Alternatively, you may find a class run at your local leisure centre. Adult education programmes usually feature yoga, as do many gyms and fitness centres. You can also find out about local practitioners and teachers from the British Wheel of Yoga (*see page 127 for address*).

In addition to being useful for relaxation and stress reduction, yoga is excellent exercise. It utilizes stretching to improve flexibility, which is an important part of fitness. And many of the positions can be strenuous, so it will build up your strength as your ability to perform the positions correctly improves.

EXERCISE

There is little doubt that getting regular exercise is one of the best ways in which you can help yourself. Exercise has so many benefits. It can reduce your stress levels, help you beat depression, keep your weight steady, strengthen bones, ward off some illnesses and disease by improving the functioning of your immune system, reduce your risk of heart disease, reduce the signs of ageing, and improve your self-esteem.

The benefits of exercise are both immediate and long term. While you are exercising, endorphins (chemicals which act as natural antidepressants and painkillers) are released. People who exercise say that they feel better for hours after a session. And because exercise helps speed up your metabolism, you will burn more calories.

In the long term you will find you are stronger and more flexible, you can run for buses, climb stairs without getting out of breath, and may have fewer colds and infections.

Many people are put off exercising because they think it will take hours each week or will be uncomfortable or difficult. This isn't the case. You do not need to take daily step classes, run five miles each night after work or use complicated equipment. The key to sticking with exercise is to find something that you enjoy. This could be dance classes, tennis, swimming, horse riding or walking.

Many sports medicine experts say we should concentrate on three areas of fitness – stamina, strength and suppleness.

To improve your stamina, they suggest about 20 minutes of aerobic exercise three times a week. This should be enough to keep your heart and circulatory system in good shape. Aerobic exercise gets your heart pumping and increases your breathing rate, and can be sustained for relatively long periods of time. It is called aerobic because you must take in extra oxygen for your muscles to use while exercising. Types of aerobic exercise include brisk walking, swimming, cycling, running or aerobics classes.

Exercising for strength helps protect your bones, muscles and joints. Most strength exercises include some type of weight training. The weights could be machines, free weights such as dumbbells, or even your own body weight, as with sit-ups.

If you are supple you will be able to bend, reach and stretch without causing any pain or damage. Most exercises help you improve your flexibility, but stretching classes and yoga are particularly good for improving suppleness.

Rather than taking up one sport or activity, it is a good idea to vary the exercise you get. This helps ensure that you are improving your all-round fitness. It also keeps you from getting bored with the same old routine, especially if initially you see exercise as a chore rather than a pleasure.

First Steps to Fitness

The following tips will help getting started that much easier:

- Before starting any exercise programme, discuss it with your doctor.
- Start slowly, especially if it has been some time since you've exercised. If you rush into it you may injure yourself, or feel so worn out the next day you are put off continuing with your programme.
- The key is moderation. You needn't plan out a heavy programme – you will benefit from all exercise, not just intensive workouts.
- Move more during the day. Take the stairs rather than the lift, walk down to the shops instead of taking the car, and get off the bus a stop or two early and walk the rest of the way. This helps make exercise a part of your daily life rather than something you do only a few special times a week.
- Make exercise a family activity. Go for walks in the country, join the local leisure centre, or take dance classes or yoga lessons with your partner.
- If it hurts, stop. The old saying 'No pain, no gain' is not true. Exercise shouldn't hurt, and if you are doing it incorrectly or at too high a level for your fitness you could pull and strain muscles. Being sore afterwards will only dampen your enthusiasm.

The Role of Complementary Therapies

There is always a lot of discussion and dissent when alternative or complementary therapies are discussed in the treatment of disease. Many conventional or orthodox medical practitioners are dismissive of complementary therapies and the role they play in helping patients feel better.

As yet there have been very few clinical trials showing that specific complementary treatments or therapies can help the course of ulcer disease. Some herbal medicines have been shown to help, and of course in the East, for example in China, herbal medicine is mainstream rather than alternative.

Complementary therapies can help to combat tension, stress-related conditions such as headache or insomnia, and even feelings of low self-esteem. However, it is vital that you NEVER stop taking any medication or change any treatment regime you are on without first consulting your doctor. As their name suggests, complementary therapies are not intended to replace orthodox medical treatment; instead they are meant to be used alongside any other forms of treatment you are on. Even if they have no effect on your ulcer, in most cases alternative therapies can make you feel more relaxed and better about yourself. And because complementary therapists focus very closely on their patients, the attention to your health and well-being can be very positive, especially if you have felt unwell for quite a while.

FINDING A PRACTITIONER

Because so many areas of complementary health are unregulated by the Government, almost anyone can set up as a therapist. So it is especially important to take the time to find a qualified practitioner.

Many practitioners of the various therapies have established professional organizations and registering bodies. These will have criteria for instruction, accreditation and good practice policies. Addresses for the organizations discussed here are supplied in the Useful Addresses section (*see page 126*).

Most of these organizations will be able to send you a list of qualified practitioners in your area. Do not be afraid to ask what qualifications they require and what kind of training their members have undertaken. They will also usually be able to provide information about the therapy: what it involves, what it is useful for, and what you can expect from treatment.

Once you have found a practitioner and made an appointment, again, do not be afraid to ask questions. You should find out a bit more about the therapist's personal qualifications, how long he or she has been practising and what training he or she has undergone.

The most important aspect of your treatment is to ensure that you trust the therapist and feel comfortable. This helps to establish a good working relationship, and just as this is important with a medical doctor, it is equally important with a complementary therapist.

You should also ask how much each treatment or session will cost, and try to get a rough idea of how much an entire course, if necessary, will cost you. You may think trying a particular complementary therapy would be helpful, only to find out that it may be prohibitively expensive for you. In many cases the therapist will not be able to tell you much more than how much each session costs initially. Once you have had an assessment and initial treatment, the practitioner will be better placed to give you an idea of how many treatments you will need, and how long all this will take.

Some forms of complementary therapy are available on the National Health, but much will depend on your GP, whether his or her practice is fund-holding, and/or whether there is a complementary therapist connected to the practice. Many doctors have undergone training in therapies such as acupuncture or hypnotherapy.

WHAT'S AVAILABLE
Although there are any number of complementary therapies available, here is a brief outline of the ones most commonly used and most popular.

Acupuncture
Acupuncture involves inserting needles or applying pressure (when it is usually called 'acupressure') to specific points along the body's meridian system – invisible channels beneath the skin along which it is said life energy flows. This energy or life-force is called Qi in Chinese medicine.

Many conditions are said to be the result of an imbalance of energy along these meridians; acupuncture therapists aim to unblock and rebalance your energy flow. The Western view of acupuncture is that it in some way helps release endorphins, the body's natural painkillers, which is why it is so good for conditions such as headache, anxiety, and depression.

The needles are very fine and usually disposable or sterilized, so there is no risk of infection. They do not cause pain or bleeding, though you may notice a slight ache or tingling sensation after treatment.

Aromatherapy
Aromatherapy uses essential oils distilled from plants and flowers, often along with massage. The essential oils help deliver powerful molecules of the oils to the nervous and circulatory systems of the body, and also the olfactory centres of the brain. The oils can be added to a carrier lotion and massaged on, added to baths, put on a tissue and inhaled, or used in a compress.

The medicinal properties of plant oils have been recognized for thousands of years. Initially aromatherapy gained popularity as a beauty treatment, but more and more people are recognizing its healing potential. Smells can affect the brain, our moods and, ultimately, our health.

You can buy essential oils from health food shops and by mail order, but you must use them carefully as they can be quite powerful. And you must take care with some of the oils if you are pregnant. You can also go to a professional qualified aromatherapist, who can offer more practical support and advice.

Herbal Medicine

Herbal medicine has been used for thousands of years, and is gaining in popularity in Britain. There are both Chinese and Western herbalists, and the herbs they use (as well as their diagnostic techniques) will differ. They may also have different ideas about the cause of your symptoms.

Herbalism seeks to restore the body's ability to heal itself, physically, mentally and emotionally. Herbalists will not generally treat symptoms in isolation. Most herbalists will ask a number of questions about your lifestyle, for instance whether or not you smoke, what your diet is like, whether you take exercise, and what your emotional state is at present. Traditional Chinese herbalists will often look at your tongue, as they believe that the tongue is a good barometer of health. Both Western and Chinese herbalists may also give you a simple physical examination as well.

Once they have made a diagnosis, they will give you an appropriate remedy, with careful instructions on how to take it. In some cases it will be prepared there and then, in others you may need to get the herbs from a herbalist at a different location.

In some cases you may feel better almost immediately, although for more chronic conditions relief could take some time. You usually will go back for another appointment relatively soon after the first so the herbalist can determine whether your condition is improving.

Homoeopathy

Homoeopathy, much beloved by the Royal Family, has been with us for many years. The principle on which homoeopathy is based is 'like may be cured by like' — that is, that a substance that causes certain symptoms in a healthy person can be used to cure someone else who has developed similar symptoms as a result of disease.

Homoeopathy does not try to suppress symptoms. Homoeopaths believe that symptoms are a sign that the body is trying to fight infection and illness. Homoeopathic remedies are safe, as the substances are extremely diluted. The remedies are intended to help your body's own self-healing powers.

No one is really sure how or why homoeopathy works. Treatment will be tailor-made to each individual; a homoeopath may give one remedy for headache to one patient, and a completely different one to another. It will simply depend on the therapist's ability to match your symptoms, personality and habits to one of the thousand or so remedies available.

Homoeopathy can be prescribed on the National Health, and there are a number of NHS homoeopathic hospitals around the UK.

Hypnotherapy

When used for physical or mental conditions, hypnotherapy is much more than is shown in stage and cabaret shows. Many scientific studies have been done on the power of hypnotherapy, and there is little doubt that it does work for some people.

Hypnotherapy relies on getting the patient into a relaxed state, so that he or she is more open to suggestions. This state is often called a 'trance'. Once you are in a relaxed state, the hypnotherapist is able to give you suggestions, such as that you find cigarettes disgusting, or to ask you to imagine yourself healthy or slim. When you are in a fully conscious state you are often able to act on these suggestions.

Hypnotherapy tends to work best with people who are highly motivated to make changes in their life. Your therapist may also teach you self-hypnosis techniques, for instance if you suffer from a phobia or stress. The therapist will help you practise these techniques until he or she is satisfied you can do them successfully on your own.

Meditation

There are a number of different schools of meditation; the best known is probably Transcendental Meditation. Study after study has shown that meditation can help relieve stress, lower blood pressure, and ease headaches, asthma and other stress-related problems.

Although you do not need to take a course or see a therapist to learn how to meditate, it is often best to be taught by experts to ensure you are doing it properly. With Transcendental Meditation, it is recommended that you meditate for 20 minutes twice a day.

Reflexology

According to reflexologists, the organs and different parts of the body are reflected (related or connected to) different areas of the feet. By pressing and massaging the sole and toes, blocked energy is released and the body's natural healing powers are enhanced. This helps to restore the balance of energy in the body.

Reflexology claims to help a number of conditions, including period problems, allergies, gastrointestinal disorders, stress-related conditions such as asthma and migraine, and chronic pain.

Treatment lasts about an hour. Again you will be asked a number of questions about your health and lifestyle, and then will settle back for treatment. The practitioner will use his or her hands and thumbs to apply pressure to various parts of your feet. You should feel relaxed after treatment, though some people find that their feet are a little sore the day afterwards. It is also common for symptoms such as a cough or rash to appear. Reflexologists say this is the result of the body removing 'toxins' from the system.

Shiatsu

The term shiatsu means 'finger pressure' in Japanese. This therapy is a combination of massage, pressure on acupuncture points, and some manipulation of the soft tissues such as muscles. The practitioner will use his or her fingers, thumbs, elbows, knees and even feet to apply pressure on specific points on your body. This pressure is designed to release blocked energy from the meridians, or energy channels, within your body.

Shiatsu is said to help stimulate circulation and the flow of lymphatic fluid. This helps to release toxins and tension from the muscles, and stimulate the hormonal system. You are fully clothed during a Shiatsu treatment, and you should feel relaxed and calm after each session.

USEFUL ADDRESSES

British Digestive Foundation
PO Box 251
Edgware
Middlesex HA8 6HG
For information about ulcers and digestive disorders. Please send SAE.

Alcohol Concern
32–36 Lomen Street
London SE1 0EE
For information and support about drinking

QUIT
Victory House
170 Tottenham Court Road
London W1P 0HA
Quitline: (0171) 487–3000
For information about giving up smoking

COMPLEMENTARY THERAPIES

If you'd like to know more about any of the therapies listed below, please contact the relevant address. For a list of practitioners in your area, include a large SAE with your request.

British Acupuncture Council
Park House
206–208 Latimer Road
London W10 6RE

Aromatherapy Organisations
Council
3 Latymer Close
Braybrooke
Market Harborough
Leics LE16 8LN

National Institute of Medical
Herbalists
56 Longbrook Street
Exeter
Devon EX4 6AH

British Homoeopathic Association
27a Devonshire Street
London W1N 1RJ

National Register of
Hypnotherapists and
Psychotherapists
12 Cross Street
Nelson
Lancs BB9 7EN

Association of Reflexologists
27 Old Gloucester St
London WC1N 3XX

Shiatsu Society
31 Pullman Lane
Godalming
Surrey GU7 1XY

British Wheel of Yoga
1 Hamilton Place
Boston Road
Sleaford
Lincolnshire NG34 7ES

REFERENCES

Chapter 3
1. Marshall, B. J. and Warren, J. R. (1984). 'Unidentified curved bacilli in the stomach of patients with gastritis and peptic ulceration', *Lancet* 1: 1311–15.
2. Moss, Steven *et al.* (1995). 'H. pylori seroprevalence and colorectal neoplasia: evidence against an association', *The Journal of the National Cancer Institute* 87: 762–63.

Chapter 4
1. Friedman, G. D., Siegelaab, A. B. and Seltzer, C. C. (1974). 'Cigarettes, alcohol, coffee and peptic ulcer', *New England Journal of Medicine* 290: 469–73.
2. McCarthy, D. M. (1984). 'Smoking and ulcers – time to quit', *New England Journal of Medicine* 311: 726–28.
3. Tovey, F. I. (1994). 'Diet and duodenal ulcer', *Journal of Gastroenterology and Hepatology* 9: 177–85.
4. Cohen, S. and Booth, G. H. Jr (1975). 'Gastric acid secretion and lower-oesophageal-sphincter pressure in response to coffee and caffeine', *New England Journal of Medicine* 293: 897–99.
5. Paffenbarger, R. S., Wing, A. L. and Hyde, R. T. (1974). 'Chronic disease in former college students. X111 Early precursors of peptic ulcers', *American Journal of Epidemiology* 100: 307–15.
6. Friedman, G. D. *et al.* (1974). *Op cit.*

Chapter 7
1. Peterson, W. L., Sturdevant, R. A. L., Frankl, H. D. *et al.* (1977). 'Healing of duodenal ulcer with an antacid regime', *New England Journal of Medicine* 297: 341–45.

INDEX